CARRYING ON

Style, Beauty, Décor (and More)
for the Nervous New Mom

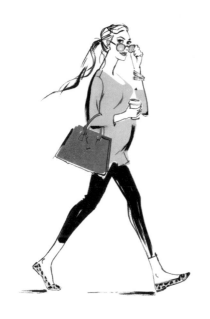

JORDAN REID

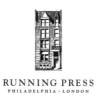

RUNNING PRESS
PHILADELPHIA · LONDON

*For River, who taught us the
things we didn't know, and for Shea,
who was just what we needed.*
—J.R.

Published by Running Press,
A Member of the Perseus Books Group
All rights reserved under the Pan-American
and International Copyright Conventions

Printed in China

Books published by Running Press are available at special discounts for
bulk purchases in the United States by corporations, institutions, and
other organizations. For more information, please contact the Special
Markets Department at the Perseus Books Group,
2300 Chestnut Street, Suite 200, Philadelphia, PA 19103,
or call (800) 810-4145, ext. 5000, or e-mail
special.markets@perseusbooks.com.

ISBN 978-0-7624-5611-6
Library of Congress Control Number: 2015935932

E-book ISBN 978-0-7624-5612-3

9   8   7   6   5   4   3   2   1
Digit on the right indicates the number of this printing

Edited by Cindy De La Hoz
Designed by Sarah Pierson
Typography: Apollo MT, ITC Tiffany, Verlag, DK Vermilion

Running Press Book Publishers
2300 Chestnut Street
Philadelphia, PA 19103-4371

Visit us on the web!
www.runningpress.com

CONTENTS

*"I really do apologize. I just don't recall
attending a single rehearsal. Line!"*

—*George Spelvin, in Christopher Durang's*
The Actor's Nightmare

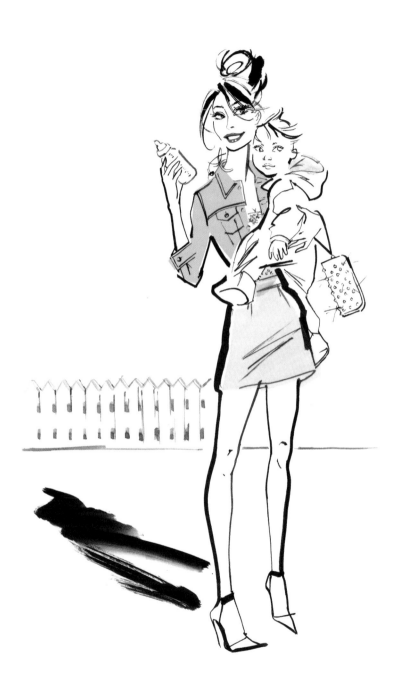

Where did all the grown ups go ?

grown-up: *noun*

a person who is fully grown

I AM THIRTY-THREE years old. I have a coupon for half off of a Botox treatment stored on my desktop, and when it gets used it will mark the third time that I have had poison injected into my head. I have a retirement account, a mortgage, body parts that are located in very different, much lower-down places than they were a decade ago, and receding gums. I get tired after a glass of wine and fall asleep after two, have no idea who the cool band you're telling me about is, and cannot remember the last time that I was awake of my own volition past 11:00 p.m. I am the parent of a two-and-a-half-year-old boy, and soon to be the parent of a baby girl.

I own a *station wagon*, for god's sake. Unironically.

I am truly, officially, without question An Adult.

On balance, this is a good thing: "adulthood," in many ways, signifies an approach to life that's a little more thoughtful, a little more knowledgeable, and a little more constructive than whatever came before (which was mostly a lot of poor decisions and tequila). For me, adulthood has brought with it side benefits like a desire to stay happy, healthy, and *alive* that outweighs . . . well, the alternative. My adulthood also brought with it two (soon to be three) new family members, and genuine agreement with a bit of commonplace wisdom that escaped me for many years: family actually is everything.

And yet there are moments each and every day when I feel like the guy in *Quantum Leap*, like I teleported out of a bar somewhere on Sunset Boulevard and landed in suburbia, my tube top and sparkly clutch replaced by something loose that doesn't need to be dry-cleaned and a baby wipe. All I did was blink, and suddenly here I am, standing in the center of a yard that needs mowing and trying to figure out how to make it through the rest of the afternoon in this uncharted world governed by rules that no one ever told me about. Each day brings a new mystery—a clogged pipe, a rash on the back of my son's neck, a bill for some mysterious tax-type organization that I've never even heard of—that I solve not with the wisdom I've collected over the years, but with Google.

My mother once told me that no matter how old you get, you always feel like a twenty-two-year-old. And it's true: even when I'm putting a Band-Aid on my son's finger, or typing "what is a mutual fund" into a search box so I can pretend to know what

I'm talking about when I meet with the bank lady, or drinking something with pureed spinach in it not because I want to (I do not want to, ever), but because I feel like it's probably a good thing to start doing now that my body has started to show signs of actual decay, I find myself wondering how it came to be that my life went and grew up without me.

As much as mileposts like getting married or buying a home or setting up an IRA can force you to come face-to-face with your for-real adulthood, there is nothing like the presence of an actual human being in your home—a very, very small one for whose well-being you are solely responsible—to make you realize that no matter how unlikely it may seem: you are The One In Charge now.

It's scary stuff. Because if you're the one in charge, that means that there's no one else taking care of business . . . and shouldn't things like the care and cultivation of an *actual human life* be left to someone who doesn't do things like run out of gas in the middle of a highway because the appearance of that little orange light on the dashboard really seems like more of a gentle suggestion than an actual directive?

When I was a teenager, a wealthy couple my parents were friends with once asked me to watch their eight-week-old while the four of them went out for a double date. Now, eight weeks is very few weeks to have been alive. This baby was very small, and made me very anxious. It also didn't do a ton except for sleep and occasionally spit up, but the baby wasn't the problem: the problem was that these people were so rich that their New

York City apartment was the size of an actual museum, complete with two separate elevator banks, a room wallpapered in leather with a wall-to-wall mattress covering the floor (hmmm), an industrial-size food-preparation warehouse in the basement (in addition to three kitchens of varying size I found elsewhere in the house), and two separate antiques-filled sitting rooms that were more or less the square footage of the apartment I grew up in but nevertheless appeared to go completely unused.

I had been planning to stay on the baby's floor (that is correct: the baby had a floor), but then I got thirsty. So I packed the baby into a portable infant seat along with a bottle and a bunch of burp cloths and toys, went off in search of a soda—and got lost. For a length of time that quickly went from funny to scary to so weird that it should probably have turned into a sci-fi movie in which Nervous Blonde Babysitter Carrying Baby stumbles upon a time-travel portal that beams her back into the 1800s, where she finds herself a housewife responsible for the care of three screaming children and the upkeep of a drafty colonial house and learns valuable lessons about What It Means To Be Responsible. Or something.

What actually ended up happening was that I got sick of trying to retrace my steps, and gave up. The baby and I hung out in the Leather Room and watched *Party of Five* until I got bored and decided to resume my search. Many turns and dead ends later, I found the baby's room on floor five (accessed via Elevator Bank Two), where I stayed put until the parents returned, at which point

I pretended that I had been sitting right there in that very spot the entire time. ("Leather wallpaper? What leather wallpaper?")

There was a moment, though, when I was lugging the carrier down a long, gold-wallpapered hallway toward what I was sure would turn out to be the nursery . . . and I suddenly wanted very, very badly to stop. The baby was wailing, the carrier weighed eight thousand pounds, I was sweating and exhausted and hearing strange noises and spotting dark corners everywhere, and I just wanted to go home and get into my own bed and read an *Archie* comic and not have to be The One In Charge for one more second.

Being a parent can feel like that from time to time: like you're just a teenager who teleported into a maze of a mansion filled with grown-up things that you can't even fathom, let alone navigate, and you'd really prefer the actual adults to come home now, please, so you can go back to fantasizing about Luke Perry and not have to think about things like feeding times and bottle warmers and diaper changes and when was the last time the baby pooped and what did it look like and do you need to call the pediatrician again. But those actual adults never do show up, and you never do get a break. Not for a single second, and not for a long, long time. Every minute of every day, it is you who has to lug that carrier down hallway after hallway, and sometimes it can feel like you're headed in the completely wrong direction and you'll never be able to find your way back.

When you find out that you're pregnant, you might be like me—someone whose understanding of what pregnancy and parenthood is like is mostly based on *Look Who's Talking*. You might be the first of your friends to start a family, or you might be surrounded by experienced mothers willing to offer thousands of pieces of advice that all effectively cancel each other out. You might not consider "maternal" to be particularly high on the list of personal qualities you would ascribe to yourself. You might, if you're being totally honest, not even really like hanging out with kids.

You might be nervous. I certainly was, mostly because I didn't know *anything*, and I wanted to know it all. Right now.

I wanted to know where to spend my money and where to save it. I wanted to know how to pick a great name and how to fit a nursery into my one-bedroom apartment. I wanted to know what that horrifying-sounding thing called the Mask of Pregnancy was, and whether my friendships and my marriage would be able to withstand the enormous change that was about to upend my life.

Most of all, though, was this: I wanted to know if all the crazy, overwhelming things I was feeling—frustrated with my husband, disconnected from the baby living inside of me, nervous that I wouldn't be able to balance my career obligations with my family responsibilities, scared that our lives were going to change so much that we wouldn't even be able to recognize them anymore, and terrified that I was simply not a real grown-up who would be capable of doing something as impossible-sounding as "parenting" at all—were okay, or whether they meant that I was really not up to the task that I was about to take on whether I liked it or not.

There is a Christopher Durang play called *The Actor's*

Nightmare, in which the main character suddenly awakens to find himself being thrust onto a stage and told to play a part for which he doesn't know the lines. Being a parent can feel like that—like the world suddenly expects you to operate according to a script that you never learned, to step onto a stage and expertly perform a role you weren't ready to play.

What I'm here to tell you is that "ready" is subjective. "Ready" is an idea, an illusion; what people tell themselves they are to make the uncertain future feel less frightening. It's also not especially important, because far more valuable than being ready to become a parent is being willing to accept that you can never truly be ready at all.

Of course, go ahead and set up the nursery, prewash the clothes, hang the mobile, read the books, and make the lists. All of these things are not only good to do—they're fun, and they can help you feel more stable when your world is about to unsteady itself for a good long time. But most of all, know this: there are moments on the horizon that you will not be able to see coming, and that will defy even your most diligent efforts at preparation. And those are going to be the ones that will help you close up the map and walk straight into the adventure.

A grown-up—and a parent—as it turns out, is nothing more than that person you see in the mirror: someone who is capable, and overwhelmed, and smart and flawed and scared sometimes, and who may not be fully grown at all—but who's brave enough to keep on growing anyway.

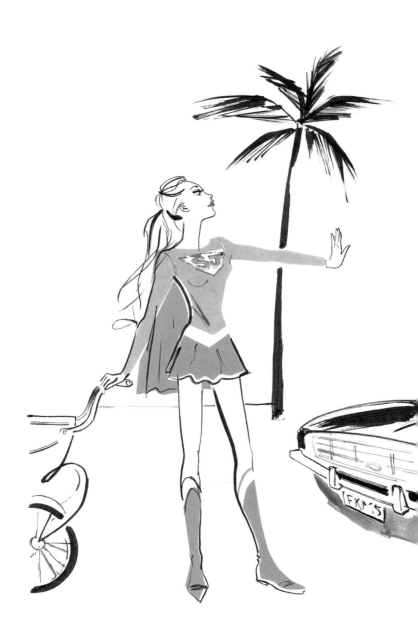

Ch-Ch-Changes

✳

What Super-Jordan Wished She'd Known

MANY YEARS AGO, I lived in Los Angeles and was broke. I didn't *appear* especially broke, I don't think. I lived in a pretty, bright-yellow house with green Adirondack chairs sitting on the front porch and drove a red convertible. But let me assure you: broke. Because I was an actress, which means that I was a bartender, and the bar that I worked at was located in the Valley and not especially well attended, and because at that particular juncture in my life 100 percent of the money that I did manage to bring in (that wasn't being allocated toward rent and gas for the aforementioned convertible) was being siphoned directly into Coffee Bean & Tea Leaf and Forever 21.

Priorities.

When you have relatively limited cash flow and are relatively young and healthy, it is easy to rationalize not saving money on things like health insurance. You cannot even begin to conceive of what might happen to you that would result in things like ambulance trips or hospital stays, because let's get serious: you're pretty much invincible, and that's just a fact.

Another fact: when you live in Los Angeles you see car accidents constantly. You would think this would instill in residents—especially residents of the less-than-great driver sort—something akin to the fear of God, but I had developed this elaborate fantasy in which my car would begin to spin across the highway on a collision course with a car coming in the opposite direction, and the adrenaline would cause my senses to suddenly heighten to the point where time would slow down, enabling me to deploy previously undiscovered lightning-quick reflexes and propel my body toward the non-crashing side of the car before vaulting nimbly out a window, at which point I would roll on the ground like G.I. Jane, ending up flat on my feet and cool as a cucumber, save for a slight air of (sexy, of course) dishevelment.

Incidentally, I have been in several motor vehicle accidents in my life (see: less-than-great driver), and while most of them panned out in extremely scary ways that unfortunately did not involve the slowing down of the space-time continuum or otherwise enable me to test out my SuperJordan powers, there was one time that actually sort of did. I was in London, where I was enrolled in a study abroad program, and I crossed the street looking the American Way—that is, the incorrect way—and was hit by a large black car. I was thrown up onto the roof of the car, rolled off of it sideways, and landed on my back in the middle of the street, but had barely touched the pavement before I bounced back upright (superpowers!) screaming "*I am okay!*" (I did this rather than do what I think I would ordinarily do in a hit-by-a-car situation—which is milk it for every ounce of sympathy possible—partially because I was mortified and partially to de-heart-attack-ify my friends, who were standing frozen and open-mouthed a few feet away, having just watched me do my best Raggedy Ann impression while flying through the air.)

So there was some precedent for my G.I. Jane fantasy. Not much, but some.

Anyway, there was a pretty good chunk of time in my twenties when I didn't have health insurance, both because I lack foresight and because I honestly never would have anticipated what would happen next, which would be that my disinterest in exercise, less-than-healthy eating habits, and early-morning-hours-focused lifestyle would leave me so rundown that I would suddenly develop simultaneous cases of bronchitis and sinusitis so severe that I would actually *break a rib* while coughing.

Have you ever broken a rib?

It sucks so very much, I cannot even tell you. It doesn't

sound like it should hurt that much—I mean, some people get ribs *removed*, how big of a deal can they be?—but think of it this way: you know how you're not supposed to move broken bones? Well, ribs move every time that you breathe. Which is a lot of times. All of the times, actually.

A few seconds after I coughed explosively, felt something crack in my side, and fell on the floor, my friend Heather came walking through my front door and discovered me flat on my back in my kitchen in so much pain that I was unable to explain to her what, exactly, all the writhing was about. Surprisingly, she did not accuse me of being dramatic and head to my refrigerator to see if I had any pie (which would have been a reasonable response, given her awareness of my propensity for hyperbole), but actually did what people with non-histrionic friends do: she grabbed her cell phone from her purse and dialed 911.

Guess what happened next? I rediscovered the ability to move and to speak. And used my newfound abilities to charge toward her yelling the words "HANG UP THE PHONE," because far less important than the crippling—and, for all I knew, lung-poking and life-threatening—pain in my side was the huge, flashing red sign in my head that said AMBULANCES ARE REALLY, REALLY GODDAMN EXPENSIVE. How all this ended up: with a Heather-assisted stroll to the CVS down the block, where I picked up one of those wraparound Velcro body-cast things, a pound of Tylenol, and a Cadbury Crème Egg (because when you are sad, Cadbury Crème Eggs make it better).

You seriously need to have health insurance, guys. Like, all of the time.

But you *especially* need to have insurance when you are considering having a baby. The good kind. Not the kind that covers this doctor over here but not that one over there, pays for this type of thing but not that type of thing, and forces you into indentured servitude for all eternity should you accidentally interact with a human being who is not "in network." Because over the coming months you will be going to doctors more times than you ever thought possible, and the whole series of events will conclude with a spectacularly dramatic affair involving lots and lots of very expensive medical professionals performing very expensive medical procedures regardless of whether or not these procedures are covered by your particular plan, because the people performing them will not know or care about the specifics of your carrier (and neither will you, when you are in the middle of delivering a child).

Also, even if you think you don't want an epidural? Even if you're *sure* you don't want one, because you're envisioning bringing a child into the world surrounded by wind chimes and gentle caresses? Get insurance that covers one anyway. Because if you make a different choice at the last minute, I can virtually guarantee you that your change of heart will not come from a place of lucidity or careful contemplation of your coverage options; it will come from a place of "GIVE ME THE DRUGS RIGHT NOW AND ALL OF THEM, PLEASE."

The Very Most Basic
Checklists in the World

. . . .

HAVE YOU EVER SEEN the Restoration Hardware Rocking Lamb? It's like a perfect storm of cuteness, and a viewing of it will result either in immediate conception, or (if you're already on board that ship) the overwhelming need to fill your nursery-to-be with retro-inspired playthings that are imported (!) and embroidered (!) and priced accordingly, and that your offspring is guaranteed to completely ignore for the entirety of their childhood. In fact, it is likely that she will not even notice the pricey farm animal sitting in the corner of her room and accumulating layers of dust until around age sixteen, when she will cut a hole into its signature (!) textured (!) plush fur, and then use that hole to hide her diary, the rolling papers that her best friend gave her, and the address of the place that her boyfriend Alex told her will tattoo you without asking for ID first.

The Restoration Hardware Rocking Lamb is super cute, as are its cousins, the Rocking Elephant, the Rocking Bunny, and the Rocking Cat. I get it; I totally wanted it, too. You don't need it. You also don't need the hand-knotted Moses basket, the washed organic linen bassinet bedding, the appliquéd-fleur, ruffled decorative pillows, or the dry-clean-only cashmere stroller blanket. (If you take home just one thing from the entirety of this book, please let it be not to allow your infant to come into contact with a single atom of fabric that must be dry-cleaned, because what your infant will do with that atom of fabric is kill it.)

There are some things you really do need when you're bringing a new life into the world. You need food, a roof, and the ability to put the needs of another human being ahead of your own for a good long while (or at least the ability to consider that as an option). But the rest of it? It's mostly just stuff, and more than that: it's mostly stuff you can do without quite nicely.

Let me break it down for you.

WHAT YOU REALLY SHOULD HAVE

Housing you like and can afford: When we were expecting our first child, I freaked out a whole bunch about whether or not our one-bedroom apartment was big enough or nice enough for a baby. And then I had a baby, and discovered that what they do for the first few months of their lives is primarily stare at shadows like they are Bruce Willis movies. A huge, spectacularly decorated house would be lovely, but for quite some time your child not only won't care, he won't even be able to explore, comprehend, or focus his little eyes on those crystal drawer-pulls you spent hours choosing at Anthropologie. Far more important is your peace of mind, and having a living space that doesn't stretch your budget to its absolute limit can do wonders for that. Besides, creating a beautiful home environment doesn't have to cost a fortune. Add color. Bring in plants. Focus on making it cozy and comfortable and *you*—not "perfect"—and remember that your memories from this time won't be of crib sheets and paint swatches. They'll be of your brand-new best friend.

A (basic) financial plan: The Good News: newborns, generally speaking, aren't the money pit that some people fear (that comes later, when they do things like walk and talk and ask to go see *Frozen* again and again). You don't need crazy amounts of disposable income in order to start a family.

The Bad News: that said, over the course of your child's life the reality is that they will cost you an obscene and unimaginable amount of money.

The Good News Encore: very fortunately, this obscene and unimaginable amount of money is spread out over two decades and includes things like college that are far away, which means you can put a plan into place right now to make it all hurt a little less later on.

The Bad News Encore: this means you really should make a financial plan for those faraway expenses starting . . . now. And you may not know how to do this (I didn't).

The Super Good News: people called "financial planners" exist, and you can pay them to tell you things that you do not know. So here is my brilliant advice: go talk to someone who knows what they're talking about, and don't be shy—be honest.

A support system: I went into pregnancy thinking that I could do it all by myself, and that I wouldn't need anyone's help with anything—not with emotional upheaval, and certainly not with grocery bags—and guess what? I needed help with *a lot*, because pregnancy is no-joke hard. There is no shame in asking for assistance, and taking this leap will be a whole lot less scary if you know that there's someone right there next to you.

If you are not having a child with a partner, remember that this does not mean that you are having your child alone. Now is a good time to start figuring out who will be there for you during your pregnancy (and hopefully later on, as well)—a parent, a sibling, a friend, a neighbor: someone you trust, and someone you'll be able to rely on for both small requests (carrying your groceries up the stairs) and larger ones (driving you to the hospital when It's Time)—because it's a guarantee that those people are there if you look for them.

A (relatively) stable relationship: This is a big one to remember: babies do not fix problems. In fact, they have a tendency to exacerbate them. Because when you have a baby you do not sleep, and when you do not sleep everything is worse. Raising a child takes an enormous amount of time and energy . . . and time and energy, unlike love, are limited resources. From time to time, you will feel edgy, exhausted, overwhelmed, scattered, and frustrated, and when you're any one of the above, the words that come out of your mouth have a habit of doing so wrong.

So before the baby arrives, it's crucial that you and your partner accept the fact that the coming months (and years) are going to be challenging; agreeing to try to be constructive (even when you both feel like pointing fingers and yelling "It's your fault") will go a long way. A lot of people think therapists aren't for them; this is a good time to reconsider. In an emotionally charged, sleep-deprived environment that often involves clashing morals and values, having a third party whose sole purpose is to offer a logical and clear perspective sitting right there in the room with you, playing referee, can be a game changer.

Or, if therapy really isn't for you, try this: get a pen and paper, write down arguments that you can imagine having with your partner, and work through them now rather than later, because later you will be holding poopy diapers and it will be three in the morning, and you will be both less productive and less interested in mature conflict resolution.

Every couple has arguments, and the important thing is not to make sure that you "never fight"—you're going to fight—but rather to fight *right,* with an eye toward the goal: all parties involved should leave a disagreement having listened and feeling as though they have been heard. Support each other, and you will also set a good precedent for the very small person who is right there next to you, absorbing every single thing that you say. (Terrifying, I know. Guess what? They also notice when you yell at your dogs and curse at the guy in the next lane, which means you don't get to do those things anymore, either.) You don't need to be perfect, you just need to be willing to put in the work. That's the best example you can set.

WHAT YOU REALLY DON'T NEED

The desire to "settle down": The secret I know you don't believe: you're going to want to be with your child more than you want to do any of the things you're worrying about missing out on. The other secret: it's not an either/or situation. You likely have a few months of mostly hanging out at home on the horizon, but that doesn't mean that the "old you" has to go away entirely; if going to restaurants (or to see plays, or live music, or whatever) is a really big part of your life and something that's really important to you, *you can make it work*. You just need to be flexible.

The desire to hang out with a child: I'm not especially crazy about the prospect of hanging out with kids. Never have been. But I *love* my kid—truly, madly, deeply, all that—and I love hanging out with him. You don't need to be one of those preternaturally maternal people who's just great with children in order to be great at hanging out with your own. You'll likely even discover that hanging out with your child is the most fun thing you've ever done in your life.

Also, sometimes you will be bored with your child and really just want to stop playing "zoom zoom" so you can go catch up on *Scandal.* That's okay, too. Occasionally thinking that your child's declarations are not the most fascinating things you've ever heard does not make you a bad parent; it makes you a normal person.

The Restoration Hardware Rocking Lamb: It's really cute. You don't need it.

Emotional Manipulation, Buns in Ovens, and Other Poor Ideas

. . . .

I WENT TO BED ONE NIGHT in February of 2011 absolutely certain that I was not pregnant, and woke up the next morning absolutely certain that I was. Because, you understand, I had *made it so.*

I once told my husband that I didn't consider myself a superstitious person, and he gave me the kind of wide-eyed "you crazy" look typically reserved for emojis. And the reason he gave me this look was pretty valid, actually. You see, I had told him about this thing that I used to do throughout my academic career whenever I had a test, which was take the test and then immediately convince myself that I had performed atrociously, working myself up into such a state that I often ended up physically ill from terror of the ruin into which I had just thrown my life. If even a flicker of "Hmm . . . maybe I actually did okay" entered my mind, I immediately flung it out like a rotting carcass and recommenced crying, complete with grand declarations to anyone who would listen that I had no future, no prospects. Nothing!

Why did I do this crazy thing?

Because I honestly, depths-of-my-soul believed that my success on any given test was inversely proportional to just how upset I was about the prospect of having failed it. The more miserable I could make myself, the more likely it was that things would turn out as I hoped. Sort of like a karmic payment-in-advance system.

This was basically the approach I took to getting pregnant.

I am pretty certain that I cried the night before we found out that we were having our first baby. And our second. Because, you see, that was the only way to make it happen. (I already said I'm aware that all this is crazy, but I am also aware that I have a 100 percent success rate going here, which is obviously indicative of my supernatural power to retroactively adjust the outcomes of major life events via emotional upheaval.)

Another thing that made me pretty sure I was pregnant the second that I opened my eyes on the day that we would find out we were going to become parents: I am not a porn star, and do not typically rock a pair of size Es, but hello, there they were. So I went and took a test, and it came out positive.

My next thought was of Jenny McCarthy. I had recently read her book *Belly Laughs*, in which she describes how the first thing she did when she found out that she was pregnant was run over to the mirror to see if she looked different. That seems like a kind of strange impulse, but I suppose it stuck with me, because that's exactly what I did, too. And what I saw looking back at me from the hallway mirror was . . . well, me, except freaked out and pale. I tried an "excited" face on for size, but succeeded only in freaking myself out even more, and so I moved on to a slightly more productive endeavor: Googling.

Specifically, I searched "how to tell your husband that you're pregnant." Now, while it seems like the Internet might be a stellar place to locate advice of the "pregnancy reveal" sort—you'd think you'd be guaranteed to find innovative and wide-ranging ideas, no?—what The Googles said I should do is this:

1. *Make bun.*
2. *Put bun in oven.*
3. *Tell husband that bun is in oven.*

No, thank you.

What I ended up doing: asking my husband if he wanted to take the dogs for a walk down to the river (a suggestion that should probably have immediately tipped him off that there was something afoot, since I do not especially enjoy dog walking or walking, generally). Once we got there, I sat him down on a bench and told him all the things that I loved about him, ending with the fact that he would be a wonderful father. And we hugged, and kissed, and then went to a diner and ordered All of the Things.

It was simple, and sweet, and nice. Romantic, even.

The next time that I told my husband we were going to have a baby involved fake Hanukkah presents, monsters, Ohio Walmarts, and grits. It was also sweet and nice, but slightly less simple, mostly because we were eating breakfast at a very crowded Cracker Barrel just outside of North Canton, Ohio (where we were visiting my parents-in-law for Thanksgiving), and there was a toddler (ours) present doing things like trying to launch crayons and possibly himself into the fireplace. I had taken a test that morning, and had decided to share the news in what I had hoped would be a fun and wildly original way: by putting together a Hanukkah present for our son that would somehow simultaneously reveal the surprise to my husband. Except it ended up being kind of lame, because my aforementioned belief that The Only Way To Be Pregnant Is To Be Convinced That One Is Not had prevented me from exercising any degree of surprise-preparedness whatsoever—which meant that I assembled the present during a ten-minute madcap dash through Walmart in search of anything that might suggest both Hanukkah and "baby-on-the-way." Which ultimately turned out to be:

- *A Christmas (yes, Christmas) card made out "To my big brother";*
- *A pair of bargain-bin baby booties;*
- *A Sulley doll from the movie Monsters, Inc., because despite its utter lack of thematic appropriateness, it looked like my son might like it;*
- *Lots of festive paper (to disguise lameness of other contents)*

But it ended up not mattering at all, because Hanukkah fail and random Pixar character or no, the expression that came across my husband's face when he realized what was going on was one of the most beautiful things I've ever seen.

It was also an expression of pure shock, because of course

I had announced just the night before that there was *no way* we were pregnant. I had even cried about it—again—just to be triple-certain.

Remember that 100 percent success rate I mentioned? BOOM.

THE BIG REVEAL: FUN (AND NON-BUN-INCLUSIVE) WAYS TO LET YOUR PARTNER IN ON THE NEWS

No matter how you share the news with your partner, it's going to be special, but that doesn't mean you can't have a little fun.

Nursery assembly: This is for those of you who possess things like foresight and time: spruce up the nursery-to-be (anything from putting together a crib to piling a few stuffed animals in the center of the room works). When your partner arrives home, escort them in to check out your work.

Dad duds: Buy one of those BEST DAD EVER T-shirts (or something more specific to your partner).

Spell it out: Suggest a game of Scrabble, and make sure that all your answers are baby-related (this sounds crazy difficult to me, but I'm also not especially good at Scrabble, and it's possible that you are). See how long it takes your partner to figure it out.

Puppy partner: Buy a onesie or tiny T-shirt that says BIG BROTHER or

BIG SISTER and wrestle your dog or cat into the thing, then have your furry friend greet your partner at the door. Your pet may have to deal with a few seconds of abject misery, but oh my goodness, so cute.

Hello, poppy seed: One of the most fun things about pregnancy is discovering which random fruit/vegetable/seed pod your child resembles at any given time. Right in the beginning, he or she is the size of a poppy seed, so try handing your partner a single seed (or presenting it on a plate at dinner) and letting them guess what you're up to.

Pacifier present: If you held on to the ring box from your engagement, tuck a pacifier inside and present it to your partner (complete with proposal-esque loving words, if you're in the mood).

Baby coupon: Create a "coupon" with a photo of a baby that says "Good for One Baby; Redeem [Due Date]" and present it to your partner. Cheesy? Yes. And adorable.

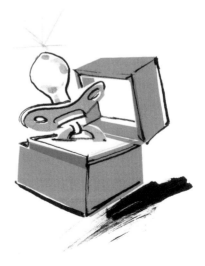

The Professional Freaker-outers

. . . .

THE SECOND YOU DISCOVER that you are pregnant, here is what is going to happen: you are going to remember that you drank a glass (or three) of wine a couple of days ago, and that you sat in a hot tub last week, and that you ate sushi last night, and you are going to freak the F out.

Don't freak out.

When I say that every single person I know who has been pregnant expressed some sentiment along the lines of *Oh my God I already ruined my child* immediately upon discovering the supposedly happy news, I am being completely serious. All of them. Including me.

Don't worry about it. I say that as a completely-unqualified-to-opine non-medical professional who is nevertheless pretty certain that the things that you did—provided that they were within the realm of things that normal people who live in the world do on a daily basis, like eat things and drink things that are things that people eat and drink as opposed to, say, cleaning fluid—were fine. Maybe stop doing them—or, depending on what they are, do them in greater moderation—now that you know that you're expecting.

But the freaking out?

Definitely stop. Go eat some flaxseed and take a nap or something; naps are much more fun than panicking.

But that's just how I see things. There are also people who

see things differently. A little more . . . let's say, "rigidly." They are the Mommy Police, and if you haven't met them already: oh, you will.

When I was about five months pregnant with my son, I went to a charity event hosted by one of my college friends. It was on a rooftop, it was summer, and everyone was wandering around in pretty, flowery dresses drinking pretty, flowery drinks. I went to the party with my friend Morgan, who happened to be pregnant, too, and when we got there we made our way over to the bar and asked the bartender to make us something festive and non-alcoholic. What we got were cranberry sodas, which are a little less "festive" and a little more "I have no idea what to give a pregnant woman; ah well, this should do," but no matter. Cranberry sodas may be boring, but they are also quite good.

A few minutes later Morgan and I were standing around talking to another (non-pregnant) girlfriend Michelle and some random guy who was tangentially associated with the organization throwing the party. I sipped my cranberry-soda, and then spotted the delicious-looking flotilla of berries sitting on top of Michelle's fancy cocktail. I asked her if I could steal one, and she held out her glass. I plucked out a blackberry, ate it, and turned to see Random Dude staring at me as if I had just tried to lick his foot.

"That drink . . . " he said, "has *alcohol* in it."

It did.

"The berry," he elaborated, *"touched the drink."*

Again: true.

Since he clearly hadn't made his point yet, Random Dude brought it home: *"And you are pregnant."*

Also a fact. What followed next, however, was a tirade of such astounding inaccuracy, alarmism, and flat-out assholery that it left my friends and me speechless. The man—who, as an aside, was about twenty-two and neither a parent nor a pregnant person himself, in addition to not being a doctor of any sort—told elaborate stories about "people he knew" who "had drunk only one or two glasses of wine" while pregnant and "had children with terrible birth defects as a result." He then took it one step further, announcing that it was a fact—a fact!— that fetal alcohol syndrome could result from contact with even the most minute amount of alcohol at any point during a pregnancy. He was positive about this, you see, because it had happened to *people he knew.*

Now, I don't know whether this man was flat-out lying, making some extremely ill-conceived attempt at humor, or just tragically misinformed, but regardless: this is an obviously horrible thing to say to a pregnant woman, and especially to a pregnant woman whom you do not know and who has not specifically requested your opinion on anything at all, let alone what she does and does not choose to put into her body.

Beyond that, I had done my own research about the light consumption of things like wine, caffeine, and fish during pregnancy, and felt informed about and comfortable with my choices, which included a glass of shiraz on occasional Saturday evenings, a cup of coffee pretty much every morning, and a few bites of sushi (not the kinds with high levels of mercury) one night when I went to a really fancy Japanese restaurant and was too excited about the menu to stick to chicken teriyaki.

So five minutes later, why was I sitting on the floor of the bathroom crying?

Because no matter how secure you are in your choices, when you're embarking on a new adventure that you want very, very much to do very, very well, it can be frightening to hear others not just question those choices, but actually declare them dangerous, even borderline criminal. In the best-case scenario, you make decisions by weighing the potential costs and benefits associated with them and then picking the best choice . . . but when it comes to your child, it doesn't matter if you're 99.999 percent certain that something is fine; any degree of uncertainty can feel like more than you can accept.

Except there's one issue: that uncertainty isn't just found in a cup of coffee; it's everywhere. You can fixate all your fears on a few milligrams of caffeine, but chances are that once you've eliminated the morning Dunkin' Donuts fix, there will be something else—or, more likely, a thousand other things—waiting to take its place in the part of your head dedicated to pregnancy worries. This is not to say, of course, that you shouldn't do everything you can to live in a healthy, safe way, especially while pregnant: it's simply to say that too much of anything—including anxiety—isn't especially productive.

All that anxiety doesn't come just from your own head, though. It's all around you: in the stranger on the street who stops you with a word of "advice," in the post you read online that completely contradicted that other post you read online, in the differing opinions given to you by Doctor 1 and Doctor 2. And it can be hard to figure out which words of wisdom to take to heart, especially when those words are delivered (as they sometimes are) with a heaping dose of judgment on the side.

Shortly after I gave birth to my first child, I found myself wanting to discuss my experiences with breastfeeding on my lifestyle website, Ramshackle Glam (where I write about everything from fashion and beauty to weird things one can do with cake plates to that time that I locked myself out on our top-floor patio while holding an infant and had to be saved by a strange man wandering through the woods, who very fortunately turned out to be a neighbor rather than a serial killer). I had planned to breastfeed for a minimum of six months, but had ended up stopping at around four months because that was what felt right for a variety of reasons. But when I sat down to write about this, I couldn't. I was too scared. I knew from experience—from the times that people had stopped me on the street to lecture me on whether I was looking too small, or too big, and from comments I'd gotten on my website voicing less-than-kind opinions about everything from what I put on my body to what I put in it—that I wouldn't just be opening myself up to "opinions," I'd be opening myself up to judgment about my parenting, and as an extension about my very self.

Over the course of my life I've developed the ability to more or less stick to what I've decided is the right course for me, saying "thanks, but no, thanks" to the people who want to tell me that my choices aren't theirs and are therefore wrong, so I was surprised to discover just how much of my confidence fell away in the face of concerns about the well-being of my own child. I was just too nervous that I might screw up, and above it all was the fear that I would be vocally, powerfully, immovably committed to a path . . . and that path would turn out to be wrong.

Part of what I do for a living is write every single day about my life and my choices on the Internet—on Ramshackle Glam and on various other websites—and opening these choices up to public discussion is a necessary (and usually welcome) byprod-uct of that, but in the very beginning, with my first pregnancy and my first child, it was just too frightening. I wasn't secure enough in my understanding of who I was as a parent—and whether I was any good at it—to let other people weigh in. And the truth is, I'm not sure I'll ever be totally confident that yes, my decisions as a parent are good, and right, and the most beneficial ones I can possibly make for my child.

But becoming consumed by the fear of failure, and the fear of judgment—all that fear can end up paralyzing you. And paralysis is often far worse than making the "wrong" decision.

So what do you do?

You remember that nobody's perfect. You remember that a lot of this is subjective. You remember that the most important thing of all is to love your child, and that you've already got that part down, even if you don't know it yet. You listen to your doctors, and to the people who care the most about you. And then to all that other noise out there in the world, you smile and say "thanks, but no, thanks," and go get an ice-cream cone, because *no one* can argue that ice-cream cones are bad.

. . . Oh, wait. They totally can?

Okay, so if they do, if they tell you that sugar is bad for you and for your unborn child and you shouldn't be eating ice cream at all, you know what you say?

You say nothing. You smile, and you nod, and then you turn the corner and go find a pretty spot where you can sit down and eat your damn cone and love every second of it, leaving the professional freaker-outers behind in their sad, ice-cream free world.

In My Belly

. . . .

ONE OF THE MOST FUN THINGS about being pregnant is the fact that all these incredible changes are going on in your body and in your life . . . but the child's not actually *there* yet, so you have plenty of time to do all the reveling you can handle.

My husband and I commemorated my pregnancies by using an Instax camera (basically an instant-photo camera *à la* Polaroid) to shoot me and my tummy every few weeks (and on special occasions, like the day of my baby shower or our anniversary) and pasting the retro-looking shots into an album, but there are tons of other fun options if you'd like to do a little commemorating yourself.

IDEAS FOR MARKING THE MONTHS

Get your fruit and veggies: Use body paint to decorate your stomach with an image of whatever fruit or vegetable most closely matches your baby's size each week, and snap a picture of your bare, be-vegetabled belly.

Shadow art: In a twist on childhood growth charts, you can track the size of your stomach each month by standing in front of a poster board with a bright light on your other side, and having your partner or a friend trace the outline of your stomach's shadow.

Build-a-Bear: Taking a trip to that mecca of teddies to make a special friend for your special arrival is really fun, and the part where you wish on a little fabric heart that you tuck inside the bear is so adorable I can't even stand it. The many, many trips to this particular store that you will make in the future will be much, much less calm and much, much more hysterical, so you might as well appreciate the opportunity to stuff an animal in peace while you can.

Dear Baby: Have you seen that Google "Dear Sophie" commercial where the dad opens an e-mail address for his unborn daughter, and sends her e-mails starting on the day she arrives, all the way through her childhood, with the goal of sharing all his correspondence with her one day? It makes me cry every single time I see it. I just watched it again while writing this, and, yes, crying. I think it will make you cry, too, and I think you should do it.

Get plastered: Once you start showing for real, you can try your hand at making a papier-mâché cast of your stomach. The only thing that I absolutely insist upon if you end up doing this is that you display it in a prominent spot in your living room afterward, because the opportunity to hang a molding of your own naked stomach on the wall just seems too ludicrous and wonderful to pass up.

Boys Will Be . . .

I FOUND OUT THE SEX of my first child while lying on a table in a Marriott hotel ballroom in front of about four hundred people. And then I burst into tears.

Let me back up.

At one point during my teenage years growing up in New York City, I landed myself a mid-level modeling agent and started doing commercial-type modeling jobs (meaning shoots for catalogs and face washes as opposed to for, say, *Vogue*) here and there. Once, I was asked to do a runway show at the Javits Center, a huge convention center that spans several blocks of New York City's West Side, and ended up walking down a runway wearing a wedding dress and carrying a whip, accompanied by two scantily clad men. Perhaps not the most appropriate after-school activity for a fifteen-year-old, but it got the attention of Ford Models, who signed me to their Kids and Teens division later on that day.

So then I spent a few years being a Ford model. This was crazy exciting and a really fun thing to stick on my résumé, but in retrospect it didn't make a ton of sense, mostly because at five foot five and more "doofy and earnest" than "mysterious and smoldering," I really was not especially model-y at all. But that didn't matter in the Kids and Teens division, apparently; what mattered was that I had a big, toothy smile that gave me a decent chance of getting cast in ads for things like cereal.

My modeling career wasn't what you'd call "illustrious," and ended up petering out when I aged out of the kids category at sixteen and started needing to compete with "actual" (aka model-y looking) models, which I could not do. So I focused my energy on acting for the remainder of my high school years, and then put the whole thing on ice when I went off to college.

But then, a little over a decade later, I got pregnant, and my hormones and my mother ("But you used to be a *Ford model*!") combined to make me think that it would be an excellent idea to call up a local maternity modeling agency and try to make a few extra bucks posing for catalogs that sold things like bathing suits cut for mothers-to-be. The agency signed me up, and I waited for the jobs to start rolling in.

Except I forgot one key fact: actual models get pregnant, too. And actual models who are pregnant tend to be the ones who book actual pregnant-model jobs.

The sum total of the "modeling jobs" I got when I was pregnant equaled One. And to call what I ended up getting asked to do "modeling" is a pretty huge stretch of the imagination, because what the job entailed was showing up at a Marriott hotel and then lying down behind a divider while a doctor from Harvard gave me an ultrasound, projected the findings on a giant screen in an auditorium, and discussed the findings via microphone for the benefit of the hundreds of assembled doctors and academics. The only thing that was getting "modeled" was my uterus. When the experience was over I went on my way with the printed-out photo of my baby that the doctor had given me, and it was all extremely weird and not even close to what I had thought I was signing up for, but it was also pretty exciting, because at one point the doctor looked at me and said, "Would you like to know the sex of your child?"

I was only about fourteen weeks pregnant, which is way early to find out sex, but apparently the baby was in a good position, or maybe the doctor was just feeling lucky. In any case, I said yes, and learned—via microphone, along with four hundred total strangers—that I was almost certainly having a boy.

And I cried.

Because the idea that I might have a boy—whom I pictured, at the time, as a sports-obsessed alien who would be separated from me by wide, yawning emotional canyons and who I would never really understand or get to know—was simply something that hadn't occurred to me. I didn't really know much about what little girls were like, but at least I had *been* one. Little boys were an entirely unknown quantity, and in that moment I was afraid that my son would be so much of a mystery that he wouldn't even feel like *mine*.

And then we had our little boy. And he is sweet and gentle and my best friend, and lies quietly next to me in the mornings eating blueberry bread while I brush his hair back from his forehead and talk to him about airplanes and dogs and the moon and stars, and what the day will bring.

All the Pretty Dresses

A few days ago, we found out that our second child will be a girl. Over the past several days a few friends and family members have asked me what about having a girl I'm most excited about, and I think the answer they were expecting was probably something along the lines of OMG THE PRETTY DRESSES . . . but that's not the real answer; not even close.

Before I get into that, though, I should probably take a minute to talk about those dresses, because hello, they are cute. Yes, little boy clothes are fun, too, and I had convinced myself that they were *almost* as fun as little girl clothes . . .

But not really. Little girl clothes are *very* fun.

Over the weekend, we went on a celebratory Baby Gap trip that probably wasn't especially well thought-out, considering that these purchases were made in preparation for an event that's a solid half year away and considering that as a parent I know that what you actually dress your newborn in are not "outfits" but rather whatever is clean-ish, but come on: tiny, cheetah-print dresses? With *matching headbands?!*

Sold.

But like I said, while adorable little outfits are nice and all, they're not even close to "what I'm most excited about." What I'm most excited about doesn't actually even have anything to do with the gender of my child at all. It's that I get to raise a whole other human being with all of the wonderful and scary and fascinating things that come with such a crazy and intense undertaking.

That's not to say that I don't have fantasies of a little girl I can talk to about what it's like to wander through this world as a woman, and who I can guide through heartbreaks and victories and everything in between, who will call me on the phone every day even when she's thirty and who will, when she is older and feeling lonely, remember how I used to sing to her when she was little.

But I know that who I'm raising is not a "little girl," but a *person*, and our experience as parent and child will be as individual as she is. I can fantasize all I like, but when it comes down to it the most important thing I can do—the only thing I can do, really—is to watch her and listen to her and learn who she is, and then be there for her whoever she may be, and wherever she may go.

So I guess that's what I'm most excited about. Finding out who she is, and where she will go.

IT'S A . . .

A child's sex is a huge deal for some people, who would really prefer to have a boy or a girl for one reason or another, and a not-so-huge deal for others, who would be happy with any baby at all. But the moment when you find out what you're having? Always exciting. Some ideas for how to share the news with your nearest and dearest:

Surprise sweet: Make a blue or pink cake and frost it (bonus points for gift wrapping it with a frosting "bow" if you're an especially talented cake decorator), then invite friends and family over and cut into the cake to reveal your surprise (this also works if you put blue or pink filling inside cupcakes). You can also surprise *yourself* at the same time if you have your doctor write the sex of the baby on a piece of paper and give it to a baker, and then have him or her bake and frost the cake for you.

All wrapped up: Have your doctor write down the sex on a piece of paper, then bring it to a baby clothing store and ask them to gift wrap a onesie in either blue or pink without letting you know which it is. You can open the gift at a party, or for a big upcoming celebration (this reveal works especially well during the holiday season).

Celebratory confetti: Put blue or pink confetti in a balloon or piñata, and pop it in front of your guests.

Guessing game: Invite family and friends to guess what you're having by dropping their names into a "Boy" bowl or a "Girl" bowl, then draw a name from the correct bowl. The winner gets some kind of thematic prize (or just movie tickets; everybody likes those).

The Name Game

. . . .

FIRST, LET ME TELL YOU that I have done a lot of staring at baby-name books and websites over the years, and I have located my favorite name in the world: Spicy. It is an actual name that has been given to actual people (my baby-name book says so) and it is amazing, and if you name your child this I think that we should be best friends.

Oh my goodness, the baby-naming process is so much fun. It can also be a little stressful, especially if you and your partner are having trouble getting on the same page (or if you have especially involved friends and family members with very strong and very vocal opinions to contend with). As an example, my college boyfriend and I once got to chatting about what we would name our children, should things ever progress in that direction, and he told me that he had always known what his first son would be named, and that it was not a topic that was, to his mind, up for discussion.

The name that he had chosen?

Atlas.

Like the Titan.

Besides the level of pressure placed on any child who is given the moniker of an actual mythical deity, there's this: I am a smallish girl, and my feeling is that if you name your child after not only a god, but *the largest god in the world* (or rather actually larger than the world, since he is physically holding it up), you better be pretty damn certain that he is going to be . . . *large.*

This ended up being a moot point, since that boyfriend and I broke up.

But my husband and I are also pretty different people when it comes to things like names: I'm the kind of person who will have a name pop into my head and instantly declare *that is it!*, while he needs to look at every single name on the planet, and think about them, and then talk about them, and then talk about them some more, before finally arriving at a decision that will eventually get changed. So when we sat down to pick our son's name, and later our daughter's, we decided to be all systematic about it, so that we would be guaranteed to end up with names that felt right to both of us.

Here's the process we used. It's a good one, I think.

HOW-TO: CHOOSE A BABY NAME

1. Decide on a couple of adjectives that describe the general "feel" you're going for (e.g. "old-fashioned," "artistic," or "classic").

2. Just start throwing out names to each other. Any that you both feel good about go on a Master List (I kept the list in my phone so that I could add to it whenever a new name occurred to me, no matter where I was or what I was doing). Consider family names, names from books or films you love, names you just like the sound of . . . anything goes.

NO MEANS NO

I think that it's important to agree that if your partner absolutely hates a name that you absolutely love (or vice versa), it's out. There are so many options out there, you'll be able to find one that neither of you finds soul-suckingly unthinkable. That said, give it time, because your initial response to a name may be quite negative, but you never know—after some time spent in its company, it may rise to the top of your list of favorites.

3. Plug your favorite names into a baby-names website to find out each one's meaning and its popularity over time.

I especially like sites (like Nameberry.com and BabyCenter. com) that offer ideas for names similar to those that you already know you like. This can be a really fun way to arrive at names that might not occur to you organically (or that you've even heard of before), but that you absolutely adore.

4. Once you've narrowed down the Master List to a handful of choices that both of you can at least live with, spend some time discussing what each name means to each of you. Try to be sensitive to your partner's feelings—if he or she really wants to include a family name but said family names include things like Igor and Butch, plug them into the Internet to see if any variations on the names work for you, or (what the hell, it won't kill you) allocate one for the baby's middle name.

5. Consider the name as a whole (if your last name is "Dover," perhaps go for a first name other than "Ben"), taking into account nicknames, and remember to plug the name into Google just to see if anything particularly unfortunate comes up (remember the Rick Santorum situation? We don't want that).

6. Live with the name a little. Try referring to your unborn baby by your chosen name for a while, and see if you still like it a month or two from now. (And don't be afraid to change your mind—even after the baby is born.)

7. Do not—repeat, do not—tell people (especially family members) the name you've chosen in advance of the birth if their opinion is going to bother you, because they will have one, and they will tell you what it is. That said, if you're rock-solid on the name and don't care what anyone has to say, go right ahead and let people know.

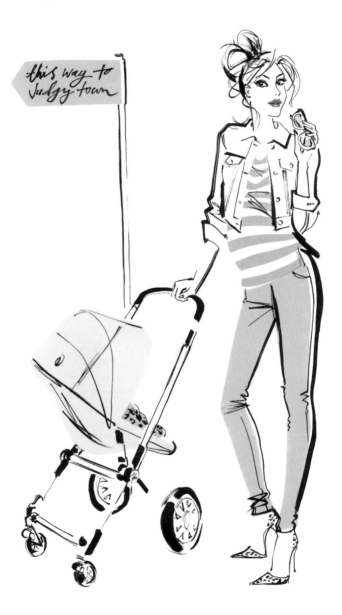

this way to
Judgy town

– 2 –

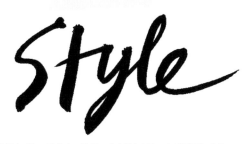

Style

(HOLD ON TO YOUR HEELS)

My Epic Flounce
(AND WHAT IT TAUGHT ME)

I HAVE HELD DOWN EXACTLY one "Big Girl Job" (by which I mean the kind of job that is performed in an office, under direct supervision, and with the carrots of health insurance and 401K contributions dangling over my head) in my life, and I was fired from it because of a pair of flip-flops.

And they weren't even *my* flip-flops.

Or, rather: I wasn't exactly "fired." It's more accurate to say that I was "gently encouraged to seek employment elsewhere." And this makes sense, because when you are trying to run a business and your employee is spending much of her days with her forehead planted on her desk blotter, the paper-thin walls of

55

her office doing absolutely nothing to contain the wailing that is being emitted from her person at a volume that does very little to boost office morale, I suppose you make gentle suggestions of this sort.

I had taken the job—which theoretically involved overseeing the day-to-day operations of a small law firm (interviewing potential hires, dealing with health insurance, smoothing over employee dramas, ordering lightbulbs, et cetera), but in reality involved mostly the aforementioned wailing—because it was the only job I could get.

After fleeing Los Angeles and the acting industry in what more or less amounted to a ball of flames,* I had decided to move back to my hometown of New York City to seek employment in the field of fashion journalism. Unfortunately, I made this decision at the exact moment in time that the entire magazine industry had a collective panic attack and decided to both fire huge numbers of employees and initiate what amounted to a hiring freeze.

During those recession years, jobs weren't exactly easy to come by, period—forget about jobs that were high-paying,

---

*To clarify "ball of flames": my final audition—the audition that very literally sent me packing—was for a Ron Jeremy vehicle titled *One-Eyed Monster* (this is an actual movie that was actually made; go look it up). The premise: Ron Jeremy's penis is invaded by an alien life force that causes it to break off and attack a group of porn stars stranded in the mountains, killing them in not-too-hard-to-guess ways. My feeling is that if your agent starts thinking that projects like this are an appropriate career move for you, it's time to start thinking about other careers (or maybe other agents).

had potential for career development, or, god forbid, made you feel happy and fulfilled—so I started bartending at Hogs & Heifers, the bar that the movie *Coyote Ugly* was based on. And then, despite the fact that the job's major qualifications included a willingness to dance on top of bars, wear cowboy boots, and throw down shots of JD, I was fired because I served someone underage. (Or, more accurately, forced him to drink alcohol via megaphone, making my firing both wholly understandable and probably legally required. In my defense, drinking-by-megaphone was sort of the bar's MO.) I'm fairly certain that I told people that I quit, but nope: fired. From a bar.

You could say that things were not going especially well for me. You could also say that this was entirely my fault, but that didn't make it any less miserable. The thing is, being unemployed, engaged to a musician who has developed the ability to survive on dry taco shells because he is just that broke, and a resident of one of the most expensive cities in the world is not a fun combination. So I did what so many of us over-educated, over-privileged college graduates have done:

I begged my mother for a job.

Two days later, I was gainfully employed as a paralegal at the law firm where she was a partner. Now, the problem wasn't that I was "bad" at the job, exactly, or that I "didn't like it" (although I was, and I didn't). The problem was that the fact that I had attended a fancy university made my supervisors (somewhat reasonably, albeit incorrectly) assume that I had certain skills at my disposal, and this assumption combined with the nepotism factor resulted in me quickly making the leap from temporary paralegal to legal administrator: a position where I was actually responsible for managing an entire contingent of employees, all of whom were significantly older than me and significantly more experienced at virtually everything I was supposed to be doing . . . not to mention extremely (and vocally) pissed off about the fact that a random twenty-seven-year-old girl with next-to-no understanding of what her position required of her was now the one responsible for telling them what to do.

Me: "Pardon me, Janice, but it's my understanding that the QT reports for the Bumbler and Bumbler file should be uploaded to the WorldOx system under Client Correspondence, not Sales Distribution."

Janice: "Those aren't QT reports and I have no idea what you're talking about."

Me: "Well done, carry on then."

I don't blame them for hating me. I would have hated me, too.

It wasn't that I *wanted* to tell them what to do. I seriously did not. Ever. Except my job description was quite literally "tell people what to do." When my direct supervisor, the company's senior partner, had something that he wanted them to do, he told me, and my job was to tell them.

The flip-flops were my breaking point.

One day, in the very hottest part of a New York City summer (which can be very, very hot), I was called into my boss's office and informed that I was to send out an e-mail educating the staff of the law firm on appropriate footwear. It turned out that a bunch of people had been spotted wearing flip-flops around the office, which was understandable (like I said: hot), but also not really the best thing to be wearing when one encounters an important client wandering down the hallway.

"Sure," I said. "I can do that." No big deal, right?

Except had I given this matter one additional iota of thought, I would have stumbled across a minor problem: in addition to the many other qualities that made me not especially well suited to that particular path of employment, I was also a catastrophically inappropriate dresser.

I'm serious. The things I wore were not okay. I mean, it was a *law firm*, and I rolled into work in the mornings wearing everything from dresses that hit at mid-thigh (and may actually have been more accurately called "shirts") to very definitely not opaque blouses to—tragically—numerous pairs of open-toed sandals that might not have qualified as "flip-flops," per se, but most certainly came back to haunt me in the hours after I sent out an e-mail to the staff informing them that they were no longer permitted to wear flip-flops, and received a series of reply e-mails that referenced my own footwear choices in rather strong language. These reply e-mails also informed me that I had a Napoleon complex, that the support staff would not be receiving instruction from me on a topic on which I was sorely unqualified to opine, and that I was a ho-bag.

Fair enough.

Time to go.

At the end of that day I went into my boss's office and did something that felt at the time like "quitting" (and that I definitely referred to as such in the self-righteous recaps that I delivered to anyone who would listen in the days that followed), but that, upon reflection, I actually think bore a much closer resemblance to the aforementioned firing (aka "gentle encouragement to go elsewhere").

Me: <wailing to boss> "I have to *leaaaaave.*"

Boss: "That sounds like a good idea."

Me: "I'm just so *unhaaaaappy.*"

Boss: "Seriously, no problem, you should probably totally go. Definitely go. Right now would be fine."

In any case, I left, and while unemployment in the midst of a nationwide economic meltdown wasn't ideal, it surprised no one more than myself when it ended up working out for the best. I started blogging the very next day, and—with a little hard work and a lot of luck—was eventually able to turn the things that I loved doing into the things that I did for a living.

At the time that all this went down, though, the lesson that I took home from the flip-flop incident was that if the other employees thought that I was dressed inappropriately and should not be telling them what to wear, it wasn't because I *was* dressed inappropriately, it was because that company just couldn't handle all my awesome. And if they weren't going to treat me like a special sunflower, I would go somewhere that would.

Stomp stomp stomp.

In other words, my reaction was more or less the same one that a thirteen-year-old would have.

The thing is, though, I was right about that job being a poor fit. I was just wrong about the *reasons.* The job wasn't bad for me because I wasn't allowed to wear the things I wanted to wear; that's silly. If I had loved the job and felt challenged and happy and energized in that position, I certainly could have (and should have) put on a suit, or a pair of slacks, or whatever it was that would have conveyed the sense of professionalism that my employers hoped to see in me, and that my employees would have respected.

The job was bad for me because the flip-flop debacle was just one small indicator—one of many—that the requirements of that position were structured in virtual opposition to my interests and values. Because it was a world in which "right" and "wrong" were absolutes, because my worth seemed to be based not on what I was able to contribute, but rather on whether I was able to get through a day without screwing up, and because: honestly? I didn't give a rat's ass whether someone had a pair of flip-flops on her feet, so long as she got her job done, and did it well. I'm not surprised that no one respected my "authority" when I told them not to wear flip-flops. I obviously didn't believe that what I was saying made sense, either.

This is not to say that it is not a good idea to dress for the job (or lifestyle) you have, or to fulfill the requirements of your position, whether you're managing a corporate office or running a household. It is. It's just also a good idea to pay attention to what those requirements say to you. A dress code of some sort or another may not mean that you don't belong somewhere, but your *reaction* to it? That might.

The things that I wore to my job managing the law firm were ridiculous, even bordering on disrespectful . . . but they were also screaming out that I wanted to—needed to—*go*. Anywhere. I didn't know it at the time, but had I just looked in the mirror I might have learned a whole lot about what was going on inside my head.

Because it was never about a dress, or a pair of sandals; of course it wasn't. It was about how the things that I chose to put on made me feel: strong, confident. Capable. Like the person I thought maybe I could become one day. My job didn't make me feel that way, so when I got dressed each morning, I put on a costume that I thought might. It's not even that the outfits that I wore to my job were such a perfect encapsulation of any of these qualities that I hoped to embody, or even of "me"—they weren't—it's that when I look back on that time I see that they were a clear attempt to convey something much bigger. Something that I couldn't ignore, and that I had to find some breathing room in order to understand more fully.

Me, I was saying. *See me.*

I matter.

When you're pregnant, it can feel like there's a whole lot getting in the way of looking like (or even feeling like) yourself, from your changing shape to your changing hormones to the fact that you cannot listen to a single word of an Elton John song without immediately bursting into tears. Your favorite pencil skirt? On hold for at least a few months, until the zipper is able to zip again. The sweater that usually looks so simple and chic? Not right now, it doesn't; it looks like a bunch of very expensive cashmere that's being stretched over your torso's new terrain in ways it shouldn't be. And if you feel most confident when you're calm and even and totally unflappable? That's a feeling that you may not get back for a while. Even those three or four extra minutes you usually allocate each morning to mini-indulgences like blow-dryers and eyelash curlers may be taking a backseat to the exhaustion and morning sickness.

But it's not the time you spend in front of the mirror or the sweater or the skirt that makes the difference. It's what those things do for your mind, and for your sense of self. It's how they make you *feel*. So your job isn't to figure out how to stretch that sweater over your new shape or how to jerry-rig that skirt to accommodate your new waistline (although those are certainly options); your job is to figure out new ways—improvisational ways, maybe—to arrive at that place where you feel confident. Beautiful.

Even though your body has changed you're still you, and you're still as beautiful as you've ever been. Chances are, you're even more so. It's just that the sun has changed its angle a little these days, so you might need to look out of a different window if you want to feel it on your skin.

When it comes down to it, of course, it's just clothing. But if you let it matter, just for a moment, maybe it will tell you something more.

The Dress I Couldn't Afford

. . . .

NEARLY A DECADE AGO, on a sunny Los Angeles afternoon, I walked into Saks Fifth Avenue and bought a dress that I couldn't afford. It was during the actress/bartender years, and specifically during a time when my life felt like it was falling completely apart at the seams. I had gone beyond struggling with the kinds of troubles that one might expect the mid-twenties to bring (drama-fraught relationships, problematic lifestyle choices, career missteps, et cetera), and had started to view my life as unmanageable in a way that felt permanent.

It seemed, at the time, like the way that things were was the way that they always would be, and for a while—a year or two at least—I couldn't imagine how any moment in the future might bring with it something different, something better. And so on the day that I walked into Saks and saw that dress that I couldn't afford, I bought it because I thought that it might help.

It was a black-and-white checkered Diane von Furstenberg wrap dress with a voluminous, '50s-style skirt, a pointed collar, and a tie belt, and it looked like the kind of dress that would hang in the closet of a woman who throws on some red lipstick just to run out and grab coffee in the morning, who never "fights" with her partner but rather "has discussions" with him, and who always, always has pretty nails. It looked like a dress that a woman who could *deal with things* would wear. Standing in that Saks dressing room and wearing that dress, I felt just a tiny bit closer to the kind of woman I wanted to be, and at that time I was willing to grab onto anything that might make me feel that way, even if that thing was only a few black-and-white pieces of fabric.

So I brought it home. My boyfriend at the time was an actor, and was shooting a TV movie a few states away, and I thought that it might be nice to wear it on a date once he got back. Our two-year-old relationship was not good (it was terrible, actually, full of screaming fights and wildly differing life goals and emotional recklessness and even cruelty) but I think part of me hoped that in that dress I'd look like the kind of woman worth fixing things for.

And then, just a couple of days later—before I'd even gotten the chance to put the dress on—an acquaintance sent me a link to some red carpet photos of a movie premiere taking place about ten minutes away from my house. The photos featured my boyfriend, whom I had thought was still out of town filming his movie (I thought this both because he had told me that he was and because he lived with me, making it pretty difficult for him to be located in-state without my knowledge) and a tall blonde actress who, as it turned out, was his girlfriend, too. And had been for the past three months.

So that was a nice surprise.

And?

She was wearing my dress.

No joke. The exact same one. And the worst part?

She looked so much better in it than me.

More than "better": she looked poised, elegant, successful, and more or less exactly like the woman I had hoped to look like when I bought it. Let's not forget that I was a flailing actress and that she was at the premiere of a movie that she had acted in *with my boyfriend* . . . so she also happened to actually sort of *be* that woman.

So I spent many months picking up the pieces of where I had thought my life had been headed and figuring out which direction to turn in next, and most definitely not wearing that dress, because every time I looked at it I thought of my (now ex-) boyfriend and his (not so) new girlfriend. And really, I had nowhere to wear it to anyway.

For years and years, the dress hung in my closet. And then one day, a few months after my son was born, I wrote a script for an episode of my home decor show, *Jordan in the House*, that called for me to head over to a 1950s-style restaurant and eat hamburgers (this, by the way, is a nice side benefit of scripting your own show: you get to write scenes in which you eat hamburgers). On the morning we were scheduled to shoot, I thought of my dress, and how perfect it would look in a retro diner, and so I put it on. I added red lipstick and a smooth updo, and my videographer and I headed out for the day.

And I have to tell you: stepping out my door that morning, I felt Pretty. Freaking. Chic.

Except by the time we arrived, I had spent an hour on a hot subway and twenty minutes wandering the humid streets of New York City in search of the restaurant, and once the camera was finally turned on and pointed in my direction I had melted into a frizzy disaster. My bangs were sticking out in every direction except the direction they were supposed to be going in, my feet hurt, my lipstick had melted off, and the dress, which had felt so crisp and glamorous just a few hours earlier, had sort of wilted around me. I started wishing that I'd just worn something more "me"—a T-shirt and jeans might have ended up wrinkled and sloppy in the heat, too, but then at least it wouldn't look like I'd *tried* to look nice and failed. I felt disheveled, uncomfortable, and stupid in my glam-girl costume, and suddenly I was back where I'd been all those years ago: a scared, sad girl who got in her own way over and over and over again, who constantly fell to pieces and couldn't pick them back up again. Certainly I didn't feel like the kind of person capable of running her very own show.

And then I saw my reflection in the glass window outside the restaurant, standing there on the street in front of a camera, a microphone in one hand and a script in the other. And you know what I looked like?

Like a woman running her own show. And so we shot the segment, and it ended up being one of my favorites of the entire series.

There's something I've learned in the years that have passed since I stopped into Saks on that long-ago afternoon: you don't need to have the perfect place to wear a dress to in order to put it on. And you don't need to look like the most perfect person who ever wore a thing to wear it. Your hair can be sort of weird because you spaced on reading the weather report before leaving the house that morning. You can forget to shave your legs, and be too pale, and have a wrinkle or two in your skirt, and maybe have chipped nail polish and dry feet and circles under your eyes because you got up early just to drink your coffee all alone in the quiet.

And you can still feel Pretty. Freaking. Chic. Because being totally pulled-together? That's for red carpets. It's for show. Clothing is for *you*. For real. And that dress was—is—for me.

The real me. Frizz and all.

The Nosies

· · · · · · · · · · ·

OKAY, SO YOUR BUMP'S not going to show up for at least a couple of months, but you know what will make itself known immediately? A little tummy pooch that says "I just ate a very large burrito" to men and yells "PREGNANT WOMAN AHOY" to anyone who actually cares (aka your mother, your mother-in-law, all your girlfriends, and most female people on the planet).

Here's the thing with pregnancy concealment: some people are going to figure out your big secret *immediately*, no matter how hard you try to hide it, because there are just so many "tells" in early pregnancy for those who know you best. Your best friends and closest family members may notice that you're wearing slightly looser clothing, or drinking ginger ale instead of frappuccinos, or looking a little green, or may just feel like there's something "different" about you. The first time I was pregnant, I planned to keep the news quiet for at least a couple of months, but the second that I went out to dinner with anyone and ordered a seltzer water instead of a glass of pinot grigio, whomever was sitting across the table from me immediately screamed, "Oh my god you're pregnant!"

But to share or not to share—like so many things having to do with procreation—is yet another example of something that is Your Call and that you get to do on your own timeline. In other words, go ahead and tell brazen lies straight to the faces of those whom you love the most in the world if that's what you feel like doing. It's totally okay.

That said, if you and your partner want to keep the pregnancy to yourselves for the time being, you have to have a plan of action for when people start guessing, because chances are, they will—and mini-deceptions like these will help you to keep your secret until you're good and ready to share it.

AT A BAR

- Immediately beeline to the bar (or have your partner go for you) so that you can order for yourself, and get a drink that looks like a "real" drink, but isn't. Any soda (club soda, ginger ale, and Coca-Cola are especially good) can look like a cocktail as long as it has a little straw stuck in it.
  Note: A fruit-free glass is a dead giveaway, so make sure to ask your bartender for a lime.
- Get a can or opaque bottle of beer, dump out the contents in the bathroom, and fill it with water.
- Announce that you're on the tail end of a course of antibiotics and can't mix the pills with alcohol. Sniffle for emphasis.
- Declare yourself the designated driver for the evening. This has the added benefit of making everyone love you.

AT STARBUCKS

If you ask for a decaf when your usual order is a triple espresso, you might get some querying looks from your companions. Just say that you already had *way* too much caffeine and hold out your shaking hand (whee, acting skills!) as evidence.

IN THE BATHROOM AT WORK WHEN YOU ARE THROWING UP

This one's easy: hangover. Or, if it's someone (like your boss) to whom you would rather not declare "I just had a cuh-raaazy night," blame it on the previous evening's meal (bonus points for constructing a fantasy menu containing highly specific and non-pregnancy-friendly foods like oysters, beef carpaccio, and raw swordfish).

Under Wraps

· · · · · · · · · · ·

WHILE I ULTIMATELY DECIDED to just tell my family and close friends that we were expecting more or less immediately with both pregnancies (mostly because I am incapable of keeping a secret), I did elect to hold off on announcing my pregnancy on Ramshackle Glam for a few months, mostly because I was so overwhelmed by the idea of the changes that were about to take place that I wanted time to wrap my mind around them on my own terms before I started talking about them publicly.

But. There's a little problem here, and the problem is the fact that on this very same website where I would not be mentioning the fact that I was pregnant, I would also likely be posting the odd picture or thirty of myself. And I am terrible at Photoshop.

How I handled this challenge: with about ten zillion loose-fitting swing dresses. I am fortunate because I favor the potato-sack-ish look in my regular life, so I wasn't blowing anyone's mind by suddenly popping up in what amounted to miniature tents, but what I soon discovered was that it's not just about wearing things that are "loose." It's about wearing pieces that have visual elements—ruffles, ruching, interesting draping—that keep the eye moving. That's where the *real* trickery comes in.

HOW-TO: KEEP YOUR PREGNANCY A SECRET UNTIL YOU'RE READY TO SHARE

Interrupt the eye: If looser cuts would be a total style departure for you and raise suspicions, go for layers and details: a pleated blouse with a statement necklace; a draped top with a patterned sweater; et cetera.

Trick of the light: A dark top under a lighter-colored blazer, cardigan, or vest draws the eye away from the crucial area. Add a patterned scarf on top and you have some excellent camouflage going on.

Focus on the face: Draw focus upward with a pretty updo (your hair, just so you know, is about to start looking *spectacular*) and a pair of striking earrings or a collarbone-skimming necklace.

Wrap effect: While ballet-style wrap tops are clingy, the ruching effect created by the wrapping (especially if you pick a style with extra-long ties that can be wrapped around the torso multiple times) is so busy that it'll be tough for anyone to tell what's shirt and what's shape.

Rubber band to the rescue: If your regular pants and jeans are starting to feel a little snug but you don't want to invest in maternity wear yet, extend your wardrobe's life by purchasing a waist-expander. Or save your money and just loop a rubber band through the buttonhole of your pants to keep them closed. (Obviously pair this look with a long tunic to hide your waistband.)

The Great Style Switch-up

. . . .

IT'S ALWAYS INTERESTING to me how a life change—a big one like pregnancy, but even a smaller one like making a new friend—can have a ripple effect in places you may not have expected. All of a sudden, Keurig-loving, sheer-lip-gloss-wearing, pajama-collector you starts drinking kombucha, feeling like red lipstick is more your vibe, and choosing pencil skirts over flannel button-downs. When I worked at a dive bar, I developed an affinity for a bandanna tucked into my back pocket that persists to this day; when I met my husband and started spending night after night hanging out backstage with his band I acquired a taste for vintage rocker tees; when I met my friend Francesca, who is Italian and thus elegant in a way I will never be, I picked up her habit of combing the racks at Daffy's in search of beaded dresses by obscure European designers. Some of these switch-ups were hits, some were misses, and some felt like natural extensions of aesthetics I already found appealing, but the one thing that they all had in common was that they were about forward motion—an active desire to evolve that started with style, and that reached into other (often unexpected) areas of my life.

I believe in the power of fashion to serve not just as a tool for self-expression, but—far more than that—to actually help you discover the things about you that are unique and strange and wonderful, and then show them to the world. I think trends are fun and tips can be helpful, but when it comes down to it, fashion isn't about what someone else says is beautiful. It's about what *you* think is beautiful or cool or just worthy of exploration.

But sometimes—as you might be discovering—what you want to (or need to) put out into the world doesn't stay still over time. Sometimes your look has to shift a little because of your responsibilities or because of your lifestyle or just because you want it to . . . but that doesn't mean that the part of it that makes it so essentially "you" has to go away.

When you're a mom-to-be you might end up wanting to (or needing to) dress a little differently, be a little more open-minded about fabrics and shapes, try cuts and hemlines that you may not be used to . . . but even so: you still get to dress like *you*. The trick is finding a balance between the requirements of your new world and the things that make you feel most like yourself.

MAMA-TO-BE MUST-HAVES

By now, I think we've established that pregnancy is an *enormously* individual experience and that there is no one way to "do" pregnancy (style or otherwise) "right." But tips are good, tips are fun, and tips can save you a whole lot of money. Of course, what you'll end up wearing during your pregnancy will have a ton to do with your personal style, your body type, your job, and the season, but these were the pieces that I kept in constant rotation from the very beginning right through to the very end.

Trapeze dresses: What I love about this style of dress is how versatile it is. You can add a belt above your stomach (or below) if you prefer a little more shape, wear it loose around the house, top it with a cardigan, sweater, or scarf, add tights and boots, dress it up, dress it down, whatever you like. (I picked up a bunch of inexpensive, loose, short-ish dresses in lightweight fabrics early on, and wore them so much that by the time I gave birth, they had turned into kitchen rags. Fine by me; they were something like ten bucks each. Into the trash they went.)

STITCH FIX

If you have trouble finding non-maternity-store dresses because your growing bump is making them ride up too high in the front, try hemming some inexpensive maxi dresses so that the front is longer than the back (or have a tailor do it for you).

Improvisational belts: Belts are a pregnant woman's best friend. But belts can also be expensive, so hunt through your closet for improvisational alternatives: anything from vintage silk scarves to pieces of rope can be tied on over T-shirts, dresses, and thin sweater vests. One note: adding both a pregnant belly and a belt to a dress may cause the hemline to change significantly (the front may ride up beyond your comfort zone), so proceed with a bit of caution or try the maxi dress-hemming trick above.

Bottoms with stretch: The lower the rise and the stretchier the pants, jeans, and shorts you go for, the longer you'll be able to wear them. Add a pants extender to the mix (or a sturdy rubber band or hair tie hooked through your buttonhole), and you'll take them even further. It's important to note that your stomach may push the pants into uncomfortably low territory, though, so be sure to wear a top that's long enough to cover any skin that you don't want exposed. Like your butt.

Truly excellent underthings in your brand-new cup size: I never understood the importance of a fantastically supportive bra until I was pregnant. A really, really good bra is life-changing, and I mean that with all seriousness. There is almost nothing that will instantly make your clothing fit better, and make you look both slimmer and more polished. But you don't have to spend a fortune on lingerie to suit your new shape: invest in a good convertible nude bra and a lacy black bra, and then pick up a couple of cheaper styles in fun colors from discount stores. (You can hand-wash your limited wardrobe each night to keep your underthings in good enough shape to last for the duration of your pregnancy.)

Cardigans, sweaters, and vests: They'll add polish to loose dresses and provide a little extra coverage in case your newfound cleavage makes you feel over-exposed. Plus, they make for a solid investment (you can always wear them post-pregnancy, too) and are a great way to stretch your wardrobe without spending too much. A bright cardigan, a chunky sweater, and a denim vest can make a single dress look completely different.

Non-gym-going leggings: Pants with elastic waists are God's gift to the pregnant, but for being out-and-about, skip the kind you wear to the gym and go for either a plain black pair in a luxe fabric or a patterned style. Tight leggings look great with knee-high boots and loose tunics, while wider-legged styles should be paired with decidedly non-pajama-y tops and beautiful accessories so as to avoid looking like you just rolled out of bed (see: Okay-for-Day Sleepwear, page 82).

Stylish flats: I am a huge flip-flop fetishist . . . but you know how they say when you're pregnant to always keep your nails looking nice, because if you're feeling slightly out-of-sorts those little touches can make all the difference? I found that swapping out my flops for a pair of beautiful metallic sandals was a big mood-booster on days when I was feeling not-so-hot. Oh yes: and shoes don't count as maternity wear, so go ahead and spend a little extra to get the pair you really want—you can keep wearing them long after the baby arrives.

Accessories aplenty: Simpler cuts and lighter fabrics can look more chic and feel more comfortable when you're expecting than fussier styles, but that doesn't mean you have to be boring. Dress up straightforward looks with hats, big jewelry, and beautiful, roomy bags (or at least ones that are roomy enough to hold a water bottle for the endless thirst that comes along with gestation).

And don't forget the sunglasses. While you may love being pregnant and feel gorgeous all the way through, there are bound to be days when you just feel tired or awkward or uncomfortable and when those days roll around, you'd be surprised what a little lipstick and some oversize shades can do.

MATERNITY MONEY SAVERS

When I first found out I was pregnant, I was a little nervous about the expense associated with buying lots of new pieces that I'd never wear again. But while I certainly picked up a few items here and there, I can't tell you how much money I saved by being just a tiny bit creative. (Don't worry, I'm not going to tell you to sew things. I don't sew things, either.)

Spend a lot: Where to lay out your hard-earned cash: on items that you're going to wear tons and tons (like jeans or a pair of black pants), or on items that work both while you're pregnant and afterward (like shoes and accessories).

Spend a little: One of the most fun things about pregnancy is that you get to experiment with different looks than you would ordinarily wear, so indulge yourself by picking up the occasional inexpensive dress or tunic. Consider allocating a small sum—say, twenty dollars a week—to fun little purchases (a colorful scarf, a cool pair of tights) that instantly give you a lift.

Shop your closet: I saved buckets of money by working in as much of my non-pregnancy wardrobe into my maternity outfits as possible. Sift through your closet for longer tops and tunics, stretchy tanks that you can layer under sweaters and blouses, any and all pants with elastic waists, and every accessory you can find (hats, scarves, jewelry). And be creative, bringing back into rotation older pieces that you may not tend to wear in your "regular" life but that are fun to try out on your new shape. For example, you may usually feel uncomfortable in stretchy, body-conscious dresses, but find that you enjoy wearing them when pregnant to show off your curves.

Borrow: There are some things that you'll need to get in a maternity cut but that don't make a ton of sense to spend money on because you just won't wear them all that often. If you can borrow items like formal dresses from friends, don't be shy (and while you're at it, ask if they have any big-ticket items like maternity coats lying around; someone might as well get some use out of them).

HOW-TO: OKAY-FOR-DAY SLEEPWEAR

One major staple of my maternity wardrobe: pajamas. Not "pajama-like articles of clothing" . . . *actual pajamas.*

The best thing about wearing your pajamas during the day is that you get to pretend that you're hopping aboard the pajamas-during-the-day trend and being all fashionable and fabulous, when what you're actually doing is just wearing pajamas during the day. Which is *awesome.* That said, let's go ahead and lay out a few rules . . . you know, so there's no confusion on the matter of whether or not you're actually sleepwalking.

Say no to cute critters: Bunnies and sheep are for pillow-time only.

Be bold: To take a pajama look into the daytime, make sure you pair it with strong accessories, like a structured purse and statement jewelry.

Less is more: One pajama piece at a time, please. Also, whichever half of your outfit isn't sleepwear-inspired should be neat and clean and resemble in no way something that one might wear while passed out.

Extra effort: When the overall effect is this casual, put a little additional energy into your hair and makeup. Bedhead is chic when you're in a cocktail dress, but maybe a little less so when you could have arguably been lying between actual sheets moments earlier.

HOW-TO: STRETCH OUT YOUR TOO-TIGHT SHOES

Did you know that your feet are about to grow half a size or more? It's so weird, and so annoying, and it's also probably true (foot expansion doesn't happen to *everyone*, but it happens to a lot of baby-having people). It's partially because of fluid retention and weight gain (which puts more stress on your feet and flattens out the arches), and partially because when you're pregnant, your body releases a hormone called relaxin that loosens the joints in your pelvis so that the baby can grow and then eventually get the hell out of Dodge. This hormone also, unfortunately, loosens the ligaments in your feet.

So your feet aren't actually bigger, they're *looser*. And flatter.

This size increase may go away once you give birth, or it may stay put, but either way: who wants to invest in a huge new shoe wardrobe? Not me. And I am going to tell you what to do so that you don't have to, either. This is the best trick ever (and, incidentally, also works for those times when you order shoes off of the Internet only to discover that the company who makes them is using a not-so-hot sizing system.

1. Put on a few pairs of thick socks.
2. Stuff your socked feet into your too-small shoes (ouch, but it's worth it).
3. Blast your shoes with hot air from a blow-dryer for a couple of minutes while flexing your toes and bending your feet, concentrating on the tightest areas.

4. Keep the socks and shoes on until the leather cools. Test out the shoes without socks, and repeat if necessary until they're comfortable.

The best part? This *totally works*, and increases shoes a good half size. Leather only, alas. (But those are the pricey ones, anyway.)

THE MAMA-TO-BE UNIFORM

Because you do not have a baby yet, and have not yet learned just how very little time you will have to construct things like "outfits" once there is a person sharing your household who must have orange juice RIGHT NOW, you may be enjoying taking your time getting ready every morning, dressing up your new shape in all sorts of fabulous looks.

Or you may be exhausted and bloated and completely uninterested in putting on clothing at all, because what putting on clothing involves is bending over, which sometimes makes you throw up (just a little).

And on mornings like those, what really helps is to have some wear-anywhere staples sitting right there in your closet that allow you to look pulled-together virtually on autopilot. Easy, practical, cute. In that order.

The pants: Here is your goal when choosing wear-everywhere-all-the-time pants: find a pair that is as comfortable as leggings, but a

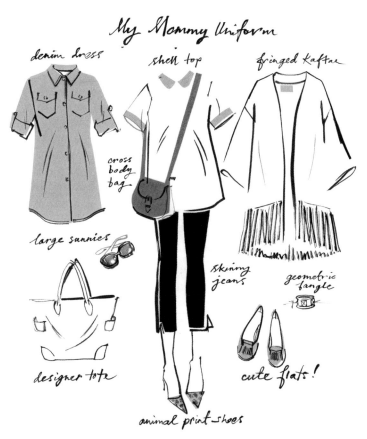

My Mommy Uniform

denim dress   shell top   fringed kaftan

cross body bag

large sunnies

skinny jeans

geometric bangle

designer tote

cute flats!

animal print shoes

whole lot more chic (not that leggings can't be chic—I am firmly in the camp of They Can Be—but I also get that you might not want to wear them everywhere. Or all the time). Look for a dark, stretchy fabric that's lightweight and non-constricting, and that hits at cigarette-pant length (midway down the calf to just above the ankle).

The top: I cannot emphasize enough how thrilled you will be when you go to get dressed and remember that you own a whole bunch of great-fitting tees in neutral colors. And there's no need to pay maternity-store prices for these: just look for tees that are cut long through the torso, and go up a couple of sizes from what you'd usually wear. Also look for soft fabric, nice draping, a great neckline (that's an excellent spot to show off some skin), and a sleeve length you love (three-quarter length is universally flattering). Bonus points if the T-shirts are machine-washable, because that means you can keep wearing them after the baby arrives.

The jacket: For a sporty-but-still-stylish piece that adds polish to a weekend outfit or dresses down a date-night look, go for either a denim jacket or an army jacket with a couple of unexpected touches, like leather sleeves or a cool hood.

The shoes: I personally think that leopard flats are something that everyone should own. But I also understand that not everyone is of this opinion, so if you're not an animal-print person, just make sure you have a gorgeous pair of flat or low-heeled shoes in a go-with-everything color. Look for one or two elements that make them unique: a great shape, some cutouts, or a delicate buckle all immediately dress up even the most basic pair and make them an easy day-to-night solution.

The bag: Go for a roomy tote in a washable fabric with a whole bunch of pockets, and it can double as a diaper bag once you transition from pregnant to parent.

The extras: All you really need to finish off an everyday uniform are three accessories: one beautiful, standout piece of jewelry, a classic pair of sunglasses, and a bright lip gloss. Done and done.

When Lightning Strikes

• • • • • • • • • • • •

WHEN I WAS ABOUT FIVE MONTHS pregnant with my second child, I put up a style post on Ramshackle Glam featuring photographs of myself wearing a white minidress with red, yellow, and blue splashes of color on it, a white blazer, and black-and-white pumps. I was appearing on a morning show to talk about my first book, and was kind of nervous, so I decided to wear an outfit that I felt really, really great in that also gave a nod to the fact that I was theoretically supposed to look like the kind of human being who would appear on a news program (hence the blazer).

Now, when you're a blogger who writes about anything, but especially when you're a blogger who shares very personal things about herself on a more or less daily basis, sometimes people write back to you. Sometimes they write words of support or encouragement. Sometimes they disagree with you, and tell you that. And sometimes they say really, extremely mean things for no apparent reason other than "Hate Blogger Girl. Must Make Blogger Girl Feel Bad" (or, maybe: "Must Make Self Feel Better"). They make fun of you. For fun. And mostly, they just make things up. I've heard everything from "you're anorexic" to "you have a trust fund" to "you have an ugly neck." Which, come on now, guys, if I had a trust fund I'd *totally fix my ugly neck.*

Anyway, I put up this white dress post. And in a comment under this post, what someone named "Ew" wrote to me was this:

"Was your goal to make sure that everyone could see your vagina? Pregnancy can be classy, you know. Can't wait to hear how you justify yet another attention-whoring outfit."

Now, I have to tell you: despite the fact that vaginas figure fairly heavily in the overarching subject matter of pregnancy, they're not really a focal point of this book. And I'm not especially excited to include references to them—and am most especially not excited to include references to my own. I mean, Jesus. But I included this quote anyway, because it's such a perfect encapsulation of exactly what pisses me off, and also because the person who wrote this sentence is correct: I am most certainly going to justify my clothing choices. 'Cause that's what I do.

So sit down.

I *love* this topic, and I love the Vagina Quote. Because it's ignorant and gross . . . and in being so, it manages to speak to exactly why I believe that clothing is about much more than just a few pieces of fabric sewn together. It's an excellent example of the precise reason why I spend time writing not only about what I wear, but why I wear it and what wearing it *means*.

When I have put up style posts as a pregnant woman—and specifically as a pregnant woman who, when pregnant, dresses very much the same way that she does when she is not pregnant (making concessions for comfort, but not really messing with the fundamentals), I have been stunned by the viciousness with which some people comment on my choices. We're not talking "I don't like what you're wearing": we're talking assessments of my attire that attack not only the length of my dress, but my very value as a person and as a parent. I've been writing about fashion (and my fashion choices specifically) for two whole pregnancies now, and as such I've been on the receiving end of more of these personal attacks than you can imagine. Nasty commentary is there all the time, of course—that's just part of the online world—but when I'm pregnant it goes next-level.

It's fascinating.

Let me take you back for a moment to a little mini-epiphany I had on this topic. It came to me, as so many of the very best things do, in the form of a bralet.

On my site I often answer reader questions about how to wear one thing or another, and one day a reader, E, wrote to me asking how she could work her affinity for bralets (the kind that you wear as tops as opposed to as underwear) into her outfit for a wedding where she would be a guest. I offered E a handful of suggestions (like pairing the bralet top with a long, high-waisted skirt, an ornate belt and a shawl for a glam-gypsy look that didn't show too much skin), but based on the comments that came flowing in mere minutes after I put up the Q&A post you would have thought I suggested she just go ahead and show up at the ceremony naked.

I wasn't surprised by people disagreeing with the idea of incorporating an unconventional item of clothing (which a bralet most definitely is) into wedding-guest attire . . . but the degree to which the mere thought of it brought out The Rage?

That surprised me.

And then it reminded me of how some readers have responded when I have worn things like short dresses and high heels while pregnant.

And then it made sense.

Because the hysteria that society creates around weddings and the attire of the bride (and of those offered the blessing of gazing upon her) is not all that far off from the hysteria that society creates around pregnancy and motherhood, which can be summed up as Wife/Mother-Type Woman No Longer Sexual Being But Rather Pot-Roast-Cooking, *Pat The Bunny*–Reading Machine.

Society simply cannot handle the link between a woman who has made the commitment to marriage or to motherhood and an enduring sense of her sexuality (which—let's just say it here—is just a tiny bit integral to the whole getting married/ procreating deal), and when she dares express that sexuality despite her newfound status . . . people freak out. They cannot abide sexuality in women when that woman's very physicality—her presence in a wedding dress, or the existence of a pregnant stomach—reminds them that this sexuality may endure, extending far beyond the period when she has accomplished her sainted responsibility as a woman: to be a child-bearing vessel.

Except sexuality isn't a lure that we throw out to hook an appropriate suitor, to convince him to impregnate our sexy selves (after which we put the whole mess on lockdown because all that attraction business isn't necessary anymore) sexuality is part of the very fabric of *who we are*. When you're single, when you're married, when you're forty, when you're ninety. And if a bralet or a minidress or a pair of heels is, to you, a way to express that very central part of yourself, that part of you that's been there forever and that didn't just evaporate into the ether because oops, you got knocked up . . . then I say you should go for it. Because for people to label that part of you disgusting, immoral, or even just inappropriate? That is to call the woman herself disgusting, immoral, inappropriate.

And that's bullshit.

There is a scene in the movie *Billy Madison* where Adam Sandler's character is being hit on by a pretty mother wearing a tight dress and a lot of makeup. The mother goes to wipe her son's nose, and then, upon realizing that Billy is watching her, suddenly starts to wipe the (presumably snot-covered) tissue on and around her breasts while making associated "sexy faces." And Billy's reaction is to be revolted, and to try to pass off this (obviously?) "undesirable" creature onto his gross, emotionally stunted friend who is at that moment torturing a young boy by spraying him in the face with a garden hose.

What this scene is actually saying is that if a mother chooses to present herself as a sexual being in such overt ways—in this woman's case, to wear lots of makeup and tight clothes and high heels when such attire is "out of place" or "unnecessary"—that choice is a clear indicator that she is also the type of person who will neglect her child, divert focus from her offspring toward "insipid" things like her own appearance, undermine her own interest in his well-being, and transform an act of parenting into a ludicrous act of seduction that, when it comes down to it, doesn't fool anybody.

Beyond that, it's saying that a mother cannot and should not be openly sexual. And if she tries to be, she renders herself pathetic and ridiculous.

So what happens when you're pregnant, and you'd like to dress in a style that is maybe outside of what society thinks is "appropriate" for expectant women—whether you're a blogger who posts her style choices on the Internet or someone who just really enjoys wearing something outside the bounds of "traditional" maternity clothing—and you notice this bullet of judgment aimed directly at you? What happens when people suggest to you that in wearing an item of clothing that could be considered "sexy" you are implicitly deprioritizing your child in favor of your own enduring interest in something as irrelevant—as shallow—as the way you look?

What if you're pregnant, and you just feel like wearing a short skirt?

Do you skip it? Do you start trying to dress more like how society thinks an expectant woman "should"? Do we really all just need to grow up, cover up, and pack our heels away in a box in the attic labeled "Good While It Lasted" now that we're moms?

Examples are fun; let's go ahead and do another one.

Let's say that there's this town. We'll call it JudgyTown. In JudgyTown, the general attitude toward mothers who wear, say, very high heels is "Why would she do that? That is so unmotherly and inappropriate, and obviously speaks to a profound insecurity and need for a kind of attention that a mother should not cultivate. Because if she were a good mother, her every personal, non-child-involving desire—including the desire to feel attractive—would be rendered irrelevant by the needs of her family."

So let's say that I am a mother who lives in JudgyTown, and that I am also a person who enjoys wearing very high heels. I go to a restaurant, and I'm spotted by a couple of girls. And imagine that I then overhear them talking about me in the bathroom, and what I overhear is something along the lines of "Oh my god, I would never dress like that if I had a child. What a tramp."

Does overhearing this statement mean that for the duration of my time in JudgyTown I should break out my mom jeans and dig a nice big grave in my backyard in which to bury my heels? When in JudgyTown, must one do as the Judgians do?

In our society, mothers are not supposed to have desires beyond the desire to have a happy and healthy family, and they are most certainly not supposed to have desires that are for nothing more than themselves. Thinking about your family should be a full-time job, and so to divert any iota of energy toward yourself is to take away that iota from your child. And that is unacceptable. Especially unacceptable if that energy is spent on something as frivolous as appearance—because then? Then it becomes downright criminal.

So it's easy to get caught up in what people think and to say, "Oh, well, I suppose I could just do what they want; it'll be easier that way." But when you understand the reasoning behind what they're saying, and then realize that that reasoning is both invalid and insulting to your very worth as an individual . . . well, I guess you just have to not give a fuck.

Because it's not just about clothes. It never is.

It's about the fact that being a mother does not take away the other parts of you: the part that loves to work, that loves to write, that loves to cook, that loves to go to matinees of cheesy romantic comedies on a Sunday, that loves to wear a pair of high heels to the grocery store just because it makes you feel hot. It also doesn't take away the part of you that wants to feel hot.

Whether you're six or sixty, pregnant or a mom or child-free by circumstance or by choice: what you want—what makes you feel great, and strong, and more confident about your ability to get through the day in a world that can sometimes feel very hard to get through indeed—that matters. So declaring to yourself and to others that you're going to wear what you want to wear isn't just a matter of "not caring what people think." It's a way of saying to a world that wants to tell you that you only get to be one thing or another, that being a mother means shutting down all those other parts of you that have been living right there inside of you for so long: "Oh, I hear what you're saying. You said it super loudly, like, over and over. You're just wrong."

Playing Pretend

. . . .

I SPENT A LOT OF TIME in high school feeling silly. Like the one people were making fun of, the one who stuttered or said the wrong thing or who had the fact that she was sad or embarrassed or afraid written right across the center of her face. I hated that what I was thinking and feeling was so obvious all the time.

Part of it was paranoia, I'm sure, but part of it was true: I *was* the one who people—even my friends—teased. A lot of the time, I was the one the joke was about. Maybe because it was simple to figure out what would make me blush, or cry. Or maybe because I was, as I feared, silly.

Maybe I was just easy to tease. I still am, I think.

Every so often, I'd decide I'd make a change. The next day, when I showed up at school, I'd be reserved, cool, unflappable. The kind of person who people needed to wonder about, who never, ever said the wrong thing and turned red and got laughed at. This determination usually lasted approximately a minute; I never was that great of an actress.

In some ways I think what I do now—write every single day about what's going on in my head—is a direct response to all those years I spent trying to cover up. And what it's taught me (all this writing-every-day) is that trying to be anything other than exactly what you are is just too exhausting. Or it was for me, anyway.

My plan, when I found out I was pregnant, was to start dressing in gorgeously cut sheath dresses. To wear things like pearls, and blow-dry my hair every day, and build a collection of chic little pointy-toed loafers. I don't know why this was my plan, exactly; I think it had something to do with Kate Middleton. Except I forgot that if there is one person on the planet whom I do not dress even a tiny bit like, it is Kate Middleton. She is so lovely and elegant, and did pregnancy attire so perfectly . . . and . . . I can't do it.

"Elegant" just isn't really my thing. I do not have Kennedy-shiny hair, I do not wear sheath skirts especially well, and pointy-toed loafers do strange things to my calves.

My plan reminded me of those ideas I used to have in high school about how I could make a decision to change it all, just show up dressed in the costume of the person who I'd like to be (but really wasn't) and somehow *become* that other person through sheer force of will.

Except I forgot something big that I've learned over the past few years, mostly since I became a mother and watched as everything around me from the shoes that I wore to the borders of my heart underwent the most stunning of transformations.

It's true, you know: wherever you go (and whatever you put on) . . . there you are.

Silly? So be it. No point in pretending.

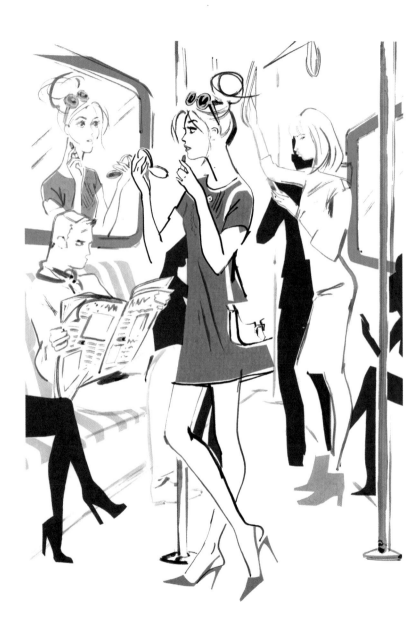

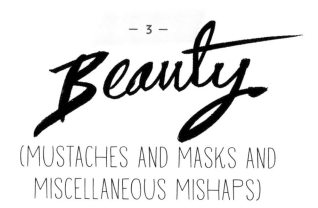

— 3 —
Beauty

(MUSTACHES AND MASKS AND MISCELLANEOUS MISHAPS)

At the End of the Day

I HAVE SUCH A SOFT SPOT for workplace bathrooms: the fluorescent lights, utilitarian paper towel dispensers, cheap bottles of hand wash and lotion refilled from even cheaper bottles of refill solution bought in bulk. Discarded bobby pins by the sink; an almost-empty Fantastik bottle stored in a bucket under the counter; the smell of Glade and spray-on deodorant. They're colorless and cold, completely absent of anything even resembling personality or style. And they're also *safe*.

They're a place to hide when you don't want to run into your boss, or to check your teeth just before a presentation, or to waste those last ten minutes before the day rolls to a close because you just can't sit at your desk for one more second and need somewhere to go where no one will be able to find you and give you a job to complete that will hold you in the office past the magic hour.

When I worked at the law firm, I was extremely—and dramatically—unhappy (and, it has to be said, ungratefully so, lucky as I was to have any job at all during a nationwide economic meltdown), and so I spent a lot of time in the bathroom. In the stall farthest away from the door, there was a little ledge that you could sit on framed by a window that was always cracked so the secretaries could smoke out of it without anyone noticing (although everyone did). I would carry my purse into that stall and set it on the ledge, then hop up after it and spend a peaceful five minutes, or fifteen— whatever I thought I could get away with without anyone coming to look for me. I'd sit there and read a tabloid, using my toe to lift and lower the squeaky aluminum lid on the garbage can screwed into the side of the stall whenever someone came in, so it would sound like I was terribly busy in there with tampon emergencies and such, not just hanging out and reading magazines.

At 4:45 p.m. every day—sometimes 4:30, depending on just how badly my day had gone and just how badly I needed to be able to leave the very second that the clock hit 5:00—I would start watching for the assistant who couldn't stand me (and who let me know it with a loud sigh every time I passed by) to make her afternoon trek to and from the bathroom, and once she was out and the hallways were safe again I would head there myself with my makeup bag (tucked inside my purse, of course, so it would look like I was conceivably doing something more important than "my makeup" should I bump into my boss on the way).

In that bathroom every afternoon, as each workday where I pretended to care about things that I did not care about and do things that I did not want to do rolled to a close, it seemed to me that I wasn't just "ending the day"; I was returning to myself. Partially because I knew that what came next was a subway ride followed by a walk down the block to a dark bar with a good jukebox where my husband would be sitting in a cracked vinyl banquette waiting for me with a beer, but mostly because of the makeup.

Everything that was going on in my life at that moment—my relatively new (and struggling) marriage to a musician who was on the road for months at a time, my crash-and-burn departure from the entertainment industry (where I'd thought I'd find at least something resembling "work" forever), my days spent with a phone stuck to my ear arguing about insurance claims and following up on overdue accounts—was disappointing in a way that felt impossible to claw my way out of; the weight of just how much I'd turned out not to be the person I'd dreamed of being when I was a little girl was crushing.

And when I looked in the mirror at my face under those fluorescent lights, I saw every bit of how far away I was from what I wanted written right there on my skin. My cheeks were pale even in July, broken out from eating whatever junk I found lying around the office and from forgetting to wash my face at night. My hair was flat, the roots mousy because I couldn't afford highlights and didn't really care anyway; all highlights did was give that creepy restaurateur client of ours a reason to slide up next to me and whisper that I looked nice today. My lips were dry from drinking too much coffee and not enough of anything else; my eyes had bags under them from too many late nights out because at least in a bar with my friends I could pretend that my twenties were fun; my lids looked washed-out because I'd developed a habit of picking off my mascara, and often accidentally tugged the lashes right off.

The person I saw in the mirror—that tissue-paper-skinned, colorless girl with a wrinkled dress and hangnails—was not the person I saw when I pictured myself in my head. Except as time went on, and I saw her looking back at me every day from bathroom mirrors and store windows and subway doors . . . she sort of . . . *was*.

One afternoon, as I was reapplying my eyeliner and blush in the office bathroom, thinking about whether or not to pick up groceries on the way home or just give up and order Chinese again, a coworker of mine—a seven months' pregnant mother of three—came in. "You look nice," she said. "Going somewhere special?" And when I told her that no, I was just headed home, she laughed and told me that it was cute that I was trying to look pretty for my husband; that a few years from now there was no way I'd be putting on makeup "just for him."

I smiled and laughed, but inside I was one big eye-roll, all irritation and superiority. Who was she, I thought, to assume that my marriage would become as bloodless and boring as I imagined hers to be—a partnership of tired eyes and frizzy buns, of ugly sweatpants and bed at nine and whatever was in the freezer for dinner and everything about the work and the kids kids kids.

I was such a brat.

I can go into the reasons why, including gross generalizations about other peoples' lives and hugely inaccurate assumptions about the link between the amount of effort you expend on your appearance and the health of your relationship (which *can* be related, of course, but are certainly not *necessarily*), but the short of it is that the judgments that I made about my coworker's marriage were juvenile and obnoxious. And probably wrong.

Also, there is this: many years later, I know what she was getting at, and it wasn't what I'd thought. She wasn't saying that I wouldn't "care" what I looked like after several years of marriage, or suggesting that the makeup going away would mean that the romance had, too; she was saying that after some time had passed there would be ten thousand other things that would be stacked up in my mind that I'd likely want to (and need to) get around to before remembering to reapply my mascara before I headed home for the day. She was saying that when I had a baby to rush back to, I'd probably want to skip the lip gloss and get to him five minutes faster. And she was right. I used to feel that if I didn't have my makeup on, something essential about me was missing. And now there is life, and then later there is how I look.

(Also: I go to bed at nine, and own a truly hideous pair of sweatpants that are my favorite things in my wardrobe, and my bun is often frizzy and I love a good straight-from-the-freezer meal that requires no more effort than pushing the "Start" button on the microwave, and the fact that all of those things are part of the life that I share with my husband does not make our partnership any less. In fact, it's quite the opposite, even though my twentysomething self probably wouldn't have been able to imagine this, and would probably have rolled her eyes at the thought. Because she was a brat.)

But I was also wrong about the reasons why I was standing there in the office bathroom with a makeup bag in my hand, and so was my colleague. Both of us made the easy leap to believing that I was making up my face before heading home—a place where, in theory, one should be able to *take off* the day's trappings, scrub away the blush and unbutton the blouse and just *be*—to make sure my husband stayed "interested," to keep our marriage "spicy." That wasn't quite right, because the truth is that it had very little to do with my husband at all; I touched up my makeup even if no one was going to be home when I got there except for my dog.

Because it was too depressing to be sad all day long, and then to get on the subway for the ride home and catch sight of my reflection rocking back and forth in the dark window, nothing outside to look at but a tunnel and some flashing lights, and have to struggle to figure out which eyes were mine in the sea of exhausted faces. It made me feel better to spray on perfume that covered up the smell of stale coffee; to pull off my tights and let my uncovered skin say that I could be coming from any of the many places in the world where bare legs can go; to apply some red lipstick that made me feel like it wasn't over, not even close; there was still so much of the day left to live.

They say that if you smile when you're sad, you feel better in the absence of any "real" change. And some say that's self-deception, and they're right, to an extent: to "fake it" in order to alter how others see you and how you feel about yourself is manipulation; of course it is. But it's also taking charge of a change in your head, and using the tools—limited though they may be—that you have at your disposal to say *sad is not my story.*

Also, there is this: smiling when you feel like doing anything but? It works. They say that it does, and they are right.

I once had a reader of my website write to me about how she hated her job and felt stuck and had no idea how to even go about starting to figure out what she was Meant To Do, and what I wrote back to her was this:

"If you didn't care so much, you wouldn't feel this way. And it's because you care that you'll put in the work to change your situation, and to do great things. And that's not making you feel better—that's just the truth."

Keeping going, searching for change, smiling even when you don't want to; it's not easy, and a desire to do it anyway—to make that effort—means something. However you express the fact that you care, that you want and need and will do whatever it takes to make sure that your life and self keep growing and evolving in a positive direction . . . that's the part that matters. I was working a job that I did not want to work at, living a life that in no way resembled the life that I wanted to lead, and my lipstick was a way for me to say—to myself and to those around me—*"sad" is not who I am. I am going somewhere, and even if I'm not certain where that place is yet, I want to be sure that I'm ready for the ride.*

Is the lipstick the meaningful change? Of course not. The meaning is the change in your mind.

Puffiness and Pigmentation and More Phenomenal Perks of Pregnancy

. . . .

WHEN IT COMES TO BEAUTY and pregnancy, people seem to fall into one of two camps: they either feel spectacularly glowy and spend their pregnancy reveling in their awesome hair and nails and can't get enough of just how stunning and gorgeous they are . . . or they feel like crap. Like broken-out, exhausted hippopotamuses who require physical assistance to roll out of bed to pee twenty million times a night, and sweat a lot, and would like this to be over yesterday, please.

At one point or another, I've had both of these states of being covered. While pregnant, I have felt beautiful and powerful and like the very best version of myself, and I have also felt like a sweaty hippopotamus. My husband has listened to me brag about the length of my pregnancy nails, and he has also had to roll me out of bed. What it comes down to: pregnancy is long, and wild, and a completely unique experience for each and every woman who goes through it. Which is also what makes it so cool. So while you may be lucky enough to sail through all ten months with swingy, Ralph Lauren–model hair and clear skin and non-puffy feet and sweat glands that excrete normal amounts of fluid as opposed to whatever goes on with my sweat glands when I am pregnant (which is madness), there will probably be days when things go slightly awry in the beauty department.

First, let's talk puff. Thanks to the weight gain and insane fluid retention (and the fact that you're releasing hormones that are specifically targeted at slowing down digestion so that additional nutrients reach your baby), you're almost certain to experience some degree of bloating—in your midsection, in your hands and feet, or in your face.* Alas, this is just par for the course (and will go away once the baby arrives), but that doesn't mean that there aren't some quick fixes you can try to take the swelling down a notch.

HOW-TO: DE-PUFF, GENERALLY

It's mostly about what you're putting into your body, so—unfortunately for those of us who want nothing but jumbo deli pickles dipped in coarse sea salt (I have actually eaten this particular combo more times than I would care to admit, although I certainly do not recommend it) and Häagen-Dazs—upping the water and lowering the salt and refined sugars makes a *big* difference. Some more tips to try:

- Eat smaller amounts of food more often to make digestion run more smoothly.
- Keep a food journal to see which foods seem to make you puff

---

*Very rarely, swelling can be a sign of a serious medical condition, so please consult your doctor if you have concerns.

up (for most people it'll be things like onions and beans, but your triggers may be unique to you).

• Put your feet up (and convince your partner to rub them) as often as possible to lessen swelling in the extremities. (Even if you're not feeling bloated, maybe pretend that you are so that you get a foot rub anyway.)

IT'S ALL ABOUT THE EYES

I have a major puffy-eye problem; always have. Or, not "always," exactly. Only for the past five years or so.

There was An Incident, you see.

I was at a wedding, and there was a dance floor situation (I think Flo Rida might have been involved), and without going too much into specifics: I put a cocktail straw in my eyeball. I am so sorry to have to share something this disgusting, and I probably should have warned you (sorry again), but this is important information for you to be aware of, because what it resulted in was ongoing corneal issues that, over the years, turned me into something of an expert in the topic of Eye Puffery.

And now I am going to share all that expertise with you, because pregnancy makes for water retention and lack of sleep (because resting comfortably while lying on top of a watermelon that happens to also be kicking you in the cervix can be challenging), which makes for undereye areas that have seen better days.

Okay, so you know how when you have a pimple as a teenager and you think everyone's looking at it, and your parents tell you to stop being silly because you're the only one who even notices the thing? For a while after my cocktail straw incident that's what I told myself to make myself feel better. "Oh Jordan," I said, "stop it. Nobody even notices it except for you." And then I found out that I was totally wrong, and everyone totally did, and all my anxieties dating all the way back to middle school were justified in one fell swoop.

I was shooting a cooking series, and as Day One of the shoot rolled on I began to feel my bad eye swelling up more and more. I tried to apply that no-one-notices-but-me logic, until I realized that not only was everyone most certainly noticing, but that my slowly inflating eye appeared to have become quite the topic of conversation. I mean literally: there were people huddled in a corner discussing the problem that was my face. Shortly afterward, a cameraman instructed me to please direct the remainder of my lines to the food that I was preparing. As opposed to the camera.

In other words: please look away so as not to scare the kids.

So we're not talking run-of-the-mill poof; we're talking a sort of major problem for someone who does the kind of thing that I do for a living.

And I fixed it.

I mean, not totally—my eye still bugs me from time to time—but it's no longer something that makes me miserable.

Ask me how. Go on, ask! It's very scientific and expensive and involved.

I got pregnant, and I started drinking water like it was my job.

I swear, I'd tried everything from fancy creams to Preparation H to crazy-expensive prescription eye drops, and after all that, it was the constant water-drinking that helped more than anything else.

It's a simple equation, really: drink water = feel fantastic and have lovely, unpuffy eyes. Don't drink water = feel bad and look like Tom Hanks's dog in *Turner and Hooch*. Up to you.

KEEP YOUR COOL

If your eyes feel puffy, it's probably a combination of swelling and fatigue, so in addition to upping your water intake, how about a nap with some cooling compresses (try green tea bags or chilled potato slices) on your face? That sounds nice.

CONTOURING FOR SUPERBEGINNERS

Ever had your makeup done by an actual makeup artist? It's pretty fun. It makes you feel very Elizabeth Taylor-y and pampered, and the moment when the chair spins around and you look in the mirror and see an amped-up version of yourself—you, but with shinier hair, brighter skin, and bigger eyes—is super cool. It's like playing grown-up dress-up, and it can be a nice little confidence boost.

It can also go horribly, horribly awry. Because although many makeup artists are very, very talented, just as in any profession, there are some who are not. Or who are perhaps just having an exceptionally bad day that ends up being put on your face.

Wearing someone else's bad day on your face kind of sucks.

A little while back, I was hosting an event for which I had to have my makeup done. When I arrived, I was led to a small, mirror-free room, plunked down on a stool, and handed over to the makeup artist. I could tell that things were going south at the exact moment that the artist started, when I felt her drawing lines on my face that didn't appear to coincide with any of the actual borders of my god-given features. When I finally did get a chance to take a look at myself, what I saw staring back at me was a woman approximately twenty years older than I actually am with Tammy Faye Bakker–style spider-lashes, Bozo-orange lips, and two brown stripes down the sides of her face.

Oh, the brown stripes. This technique, called "contouring," is very well-intentioned, with the goal of making you look like you just fell out of bed with astonishing bone structure, but the thing about contour is that—sort of like a boob job—if you can tell that it is there, it is bad.

Done correctly, however, contouring can be extremely lovely. See, the thing is that cheekbones are really nice. Except not all of us have prominent ones (myself included). And even fewer of us have them when we are pregnant, because of the aforementioned water retention, et cetera. So I'm certainly on board with the temptation to just go ahead and draw them on, but as with most deceptions, the key is to try not to let people *know* that you're deceiving them. Because if they see you and think not "Wow, nice cheekbones!" but rather, "Aw, she tried to draw on cheekbones and ended up with brown stripes on her face; that's sweet and sort of sad" . . . well, that's not exactly the point.

Which is not to scare you. Contouring can be done subtly, and it can be done well, and it can definitely make you look a little more defined during a time when you feel like your face may be hiding from you.

HOW-TO: CONTOUR NON-DISASTROUSLY

Making your cheekbones look more prominent involves making the bones themselves appear lighter, and the space underneath them (the hollows of your cheeks) appear darker. To achieve this, you'll need three products:

- A highlighter (either a specialty product like Yves Saint Laurent Touche Éclat or a light or nude-colored eye shadow;
- A matte contouring blush or bronzer approximately three shades darker than your skin tone;

- A brush (preferably an angled contouring brush, but let's get real: you're not going to go buy one of those. Just use a medium-size blush brush; it'll work just fine).

1. Start by sucking in your cheeks: where you see the lines form is where you're going to apply the darker shade.

2. Swirl some contouring powder onto the brush, tap it to remove any excess (this is a *major* less-is-more situation), and sweep the brush from just under the top of your cheekbone down along that invisible line toward the apples of your cheeks (so that the color is strongest at the top of your cheekbones and more subtle as it moves downward). Start light; it's easier to add color than to remove it.

3. Blend well. Then blend some more. Blend blend blend.

4. Take the highlighter and use a clean brush to apply it lightly to the tops of your cheekbones, just above the area where you applied the contouring blush or bronzer. Blend blend blend.

Gorgeous. Dare I say: chiseled, even.

- Apply highlighter down the center of your nose and contouring powder along the sides of your nose to make it look more defined.

- Apply highlighter to your brow bones to bring out the shape of your face.

- Apply highlighter to the center of your lips to make them appear fuller.

- Apply contouring powder just under your jawline to make it appear sharper.

THE MASK OF PREGNANCY

I love beauty disasters that sound like actual titles of horror movies; they're so *dramatic*. But "dramatic" is actually a good way to describe this one, or at least your likely response to it. Because your waddle-walk may already be making you feel sort of indelicate . . . and then oops: now you have a mustache. So feminine! So precious.

The Mask of Pregnancy, for those of you who have never been lucky enough to experience it yourself, is technically called "cholasma," and is a temporary hyperpigmentation effect that sometimes takes on the appearance of a "mask," darkening parts of your forehead, nose, and cheeks. It's the result of hormonal changes during pregnancy, and can make already-pigmented areas (like freckles, or your nipples) appear darker.

Or it can go ahead and make you look like you have a mustache.

Guess which version I got?

Correct.

HOW-TO: HANDLE THAT HYPERPIGMENTATION

Sure, concealer works, but the number-one way to lessen the chances that you'll develop hyperpigmentation (or to make it less noticeable) is to stay away from the sun. Which you're probably already doing anyway, because being pregnant is like toting around your own personal space heater, but try going next-level: high-SPF sunscreen *all the time*, hats, umbrellas, et cetera. You can also try upping your folic acid intake (yet another reason to remember to take those prenatal vitamins), as studies have shown that hyperpigmentation is related to the decrease in folic acid brought about by pregnancy.

MISCELLANEOUS BEAUTY MISHAPS AND HOW TO DEAL

Skin flare-ups: Your skin may be better than usual during pregnancy, or it may be worse, but one guarantee is that it will be *different.* That doesn't necessarily mean that now is the time to experiment with new skin remedies; on the contrary, what you may find works best is to whittle down your system to the bare basics: a gentle cleanser and moisturizer, plus an SPF-containing moisturizer for daytime (look for products geared toward sensitive skin, as yours may be especially prone to reactions). If you're dealing with acne, remember that many topical and oral treatments are unsafe for use during pregnancy, so talk to your doctor about your options.

Heat rash: Weight gain and hormonal fluctuations mean it's easy to get overheated, and all that heat may very well show up on your skin (particularly in areas where your skin rubs against itself). To combat heat rash, wear loose cotton clothing and keep the affected area cool and dry.

Stretch marks: Did you know that 90 percent of pregnant women get stretch marks? I tell you this not to freak you out, but rather to let you know that while there are certainly steps you can take to minimize these marks, chances are you won't be able to prevent them entirely, so they're not worth getting all worked up about. That said, this is my favorite pregnancy beauty disaster, because it's the most fun one to try to combat: buy an unscented oil (no need for pricey anti-stretch mark products; anything that moisturizes your skin will do the trick) and get your partner to rub it into your stomach (and anywhere else you're worried about developing stretch marks) nightly.

Skin tags: Ick, I know. But these little bumps pop up on tons of pregnant women as a by-product of hormones, and they're almost always nothing to worry about. Alas, there's not much you can do about them until you've given birth, but after delivery see a dermatologist to have them removed.

Itchy skin: There's a lot of stretching going on these days, and your stomach and breasts may be particularly prone to itchiness. If the itchiness stems from excessive dryness, avoid very hot baths and showers, apply unscented moisturizer, and try relaxing in an oatmeal soak (like the DIY one below).

DIY SKIN-SOOTHING BATH SOAK

Oatmeal soaks are basically cure-alls: they moisturize and soften skin, and can help with everything from eczema to rashes to psoriasis. Oh, yes: and they're cheap. Whee!

In a bowl, combine:

½ cup powdered oatmeal (just use a blender to grind up the oatmeal you already have in your cupboard until you get a fine powder)

½ cup powdered milk

2 tablespoons of vitamin E cream

Pour into a lukewarm bath (pregnant women should bathe in water no hotter than 98 degrees, to avoid stress to the baby) and soak 15 to 20 minutes, then pat dry.

Or try this trick: pour a cup of oatmeal—not the instant kind—into a (clean) nylon stocking. Run your bath, swishing the oatmeal-filled stocking around in the water every so often. After you've soaked for a while, gently run the stocking over your body for a light exfoliating treatment.

* Note: While soaking in the bath, make sure to drink water frequently to avoid dehydration, and have someone around who can help you out when you're done (in case your altered center of gravity makes you unsteady on your feet).

DIY SKIN-SOOTHING FACE MASK

This face mask contains anti-inflammatory and soothing properties, and is lovely and cooling. (You also may want to eat it. Maybe don't do that; head over to page 196 for my Cucumber Yogurt with Mint and Olive Oil if you start getting cravings while mixing up your mask.)

In a bowl, combine:

3 tablespoons of aloe vera

2 tablespoons of plain yogurt

4 tablespoons of fresh cucumber juice (get this by peeling a cucumber, pureeing it in a blender, and then passing the puree through a strainer or sieve).

Apply to your face for a few minutes, then wash off.

Before You Go

. . . .

MOMENTS AFTER I GAVE BIRTH to my son, my husband took a photo of me cradling him to my chest and smiling down into his sweet little face. In this photo, my hair is gently swept off to one side. My eye makeup appears to be intact. I am calm, happy. Glowing, even.

This photo lied.

What actually happened was that my husband morphed into a professional paparazzo in the face of the birth of his first child, and took something like eighty thousand shots over the course of approximately three minutes. In exactly one of them, I look like a little post-partum miracle, because even a stopped clock is right twice a day and et cetera et cetera. In the rest of these photos—which I thought about publishing in this book and then thought better of, because I didn't want to scare you—I look like someone who is in the process of giving birth, all sweaty and wild-eyed and pissed off, with a mouth open so wide that you can see my tonsils. (I mean this literally: were I to show you this one particular photograph in which I am actually screaming into the camera lens, the first thought that would come to your mind would be, "Oh. There are Jordan's tonsils," and the second thought would be, "Gross.")

Look, there are dueling realities going on here: one is that lots and lots and lots of photographs will be taken on the day that your child is born, and you will probably be in quite a few of them. The other reality is that giving birth is nothing short of one of the most taxing physical feats that you will ever perform in your life, and taxing physical feats tend to involve things like sweat and unfortunate facial expressions.

So if you have some picture in your head of coming out of this with glowy, peaceful birthing images, let me tell you now: what you're going to end up with is most likely a series of photographs that predominantly consist of you doing your best Ursula the Sea Witch impression while turning blue and maybe (definitely) pooping.

I say this not to make you panic, but rather so that you can manage those expectations.

Obviously very few (if any) women look stunning after hours and hours (sometimes days) of intense physical exertion that involves a truly mind-blowing variety of bodily fluids. But "stunning" isn't the point, of course, and another thing I can virtually guarantee is that whatever shots you do end up with will be beautiful beyond anything you can imagine.

So now that we've established that how you look on the day that you bring a new life into the world doesn't matter, can we please talk about how you look on the day that you bring a new life into the world?

Because I have yet to meet a mother-to-be who doesn't intend to at least throw on a little lip gloss before leaving for the hospital, and the vast majority of them are planning on heading in for their child's debut with a decent blowout, a nice, chip-free mani/pedi, and decently shaped eyebrows.

And I think there's absolutely nothing wrong with that. Both because there's nothing wrong with feeling better with a little mascara on, period . . . and because the fact is that once you arrive home with your child, you really won't be thinking about makeup for a while. So go ahead and take advantage of those last few moments when you don't have anyone to fuss over except for yourself.

A FEW DAYS BEFORE YOUR DUE DATE . . .

Of course, you can't time the baby's arrival to the minute, but in the days leading up to your projected due date go ahead and make time for a few beauty treatments.

Manicure/pedicure: You probably won't be able to get to the salon for at least a couple of weeks (or months) after the baby's arrival, so now is the time to freshen up your tips and toes. On your toenails, go for a gel polish that will last more or less until it grows out. File your fingernails short (long nails and diaper changes do not mix), and choose a sheer polish that won't show minor chips.

Haircut: Another place you likely won't be able to get to for at least a few weeks is the hair salon, so now's the time for a trim.

Just remember that now is *not* the time for drastic changes. You know how they say not to whack off all your hair in the wake of a breakup? Well, don't do it when you're about to give birth, either. You are hormonal and not to be trusted, and trying to figure out how to deal with brand-new bangs when you have a brand-new baby to tangle with is an exercise in futility.

EYELASH EXTENSIONS: OH, JUST DO IT

Eyelash extensions are one of those ridiculous beauty indulgences that I am totally comfortable advocating, because not only are they gorgeous, they're actually practical (or, whatever, pratical*ish*) because they basically mean that you can look all stunning and made-up without actually wearing makeup. (For two to four whole weeks, at least, after which you will need to spend another hour sitting in a salon chair getting more tiny hairs affixed to your face if you'd like the effect to stay put, but you know what an hour in a salon chair is? A NAP. Win!)

Eyebrows: Chances are that in those first few weeks after the baby arrives you will forget that you have a face, let alone eyebrows. Might as well clean them up now and get it over with.

Waxing: I hate waxing. Hate it hate it hate it. But for this particular moment in your life, I think it's a phenomenal option, just because it means that you can skip shaving during an era when you won't want to be bending over a ton anyway . . . and when you won't remember to do it. Literally the *last* thing on my mind when my son was a newborn was the hair on my legs. (Three years later, it's still pretty much the last thing on my mind, but that's another story.) One note: your skin may be especially sensitive right now, so consider having your aesthetician do a patch test before going all-in.

WHAT TO BRING TO THE HOSPITAL

You already know to bring the car seat and something for the baby to wear home, so instead of practicalities, let's talk about the stuff that you don't technically "need," but that may make the experience a whole lot more enjoyable.

Cute pajamas. And slippers. And a robe: I wanted to wear a pretty nightgown for the delivery itself and was talked out of it by my mother, who accurately (and annoyingly) insisted that it was a waste to spend money on something that would possibly end up being cut off of my body and that would certainly end up being wrecked. Where I would not bend: my desire to have cute pajamas to wear for the remainder of my hospital stay. Go for a pair with (very) loose bottoms—you won't want anything even the slightest bit clingy, and will be wearing something akin to a diaper underneath them for the first couple of days postpartum—and a button-down top (for breastfeeding), and make sure you choose

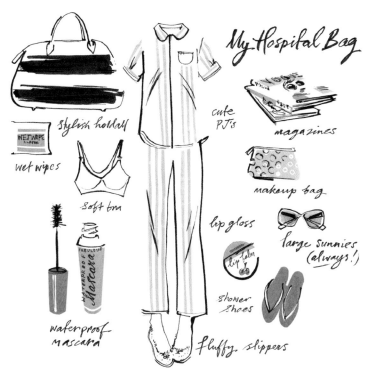

My Hospital Bag

stylish holdall

wet wipes

soft bra

waterproof mascara

cute PJ's

lip gloss

lip balm

shower shoes

fluffy slippers

magazines

makeup bag

large sunnies (always!)

a dark, non-stain-showing color. Also bring a robe and slippers for those trips to and from the bathroom, because hospital wards can be cold, and just-had-a-baby you will be slow.

WHAT NOT TO BRING

Any items of clothing so beloved that you would cry were they to be destroyed beyond recognition. They may be destroyed beyond recognition. Don't cry.

Something fun to do/watch/read: After you arrive at the hospital you may have quite a few surprisingly boring hours ahead of you. But this is not the time for *Great Expectations*. Think *US Weekly*, not Shakespeare. (I brought an iPad and watched *The Walking Dead*, which is perhaps not the most reassuring pick when you are about to give birth to new life, but whatever: I love it. Bring what you love.)

A notepad (or baby journal) and pen: During the hours we spent in the delivery ward, my husband jotted notes about what was going on—what I was saying, what he was thinking about, who was there—and that transcript has become one of my most treasured possessions. However you prefer to record the time (photos and videos also work, of course), it's so nice to have an in-the-moment account of an experience that can end up feeling like a big old blur afterward.

Refreshing face spray or wipes: You may not be quite up for a full-on washing session for a couple of hours (or even days), and a spray bottle of rosewater or some cleansing wipes will make you feel like an actual human being capable of actual human interaction in seconds.

Food: You will probably not be allowed to eat the food that you bring into the hospital before you give birth, and this will make you sad. But afterward, you might want to ingest substances other than hospital-issue applesauce, and this is when you will be pretty psyched to remember the tin of brownies or bag of fresh fruit that you so thoughtfully packed for yourself. And then you will find out that your partner already ate it, and be sad again. And then you will have the leverage required to demand that he or she immediately go out and procure you some Chinese food, and that will be awesome.

Granny panties: The hospital will provide you with giant fishing nets to wear over the giant pads they will also give you to wear (it's as attractive as it sounds). If you like giant fishing nets, great. If you don't, it's nice to have some (oversize) options. I love me some granny panties. (Just be aware that they may end up in the trash, so don't spend a fortune on them.)

HOW-TO: HOSPITAL MAKEUP

The goal isn't to look airbrushed within an inch of your life, all false eyelashes and bronzer and glossy lips; it's to look healthy and glowy and like you just took an exuberant jog through a park rather than completed a full-on triathlon. Really, what you're going for is sweat/dishevelment management, not a photo-shoot-ready face. In other words: less "made-up" than . . . calmed down.

1. Your face makeup is going to come off, and a river of foundation coursing down your cheeks is not a good look on anyone. Choose a waterproof concealer and apply it only where you absolutely must.

2. If you choose to forego the wonder that is eyelash extensions,

just go for a couple of coats of waterproof mascara; anything else will end up firmly planted underneath your eyes, and this look is only cute on raccoons. No eye shadow. No eyeliner. Keep it basic.

3. If you really want color on your lips, go for a long-wearing lip stain like Benetint (which you can also use on your cheeks), and keep a lip balm with you in the delivery room, if you're allowed. At some point, they'll tell you that you're no longer allowed to drink water, and you will turn into a furious crocodile. There was a point during my son's birth when things were getting really real and I loved my ChapStick more than I loved my husband.

The Skin You're In

. . . .

WHEN YOU WRITE ABOUT the subject of beauty, you make some people angry. Lipstick and mascara may seem like harmless subjects, but they also have the potential to spark conflict about whether concerns as flighty as the state of a manicure detract from more pertinent matters: your job, your family, the "real stuff" of life.

Is it okay to care about what you look like, when there are so many other things worth caring about?

When you write about the subject of beauty and pair it

with the subject of motherhood, you make some people *furious*. What place, they argue, do long-lasting lipsticks and waterproof concealers have taking up space in your mind and in your day when there are bigger things to worry about? Things like new life, and raising a human being from infancy to adulthood, and teaching him or her about compassion, and wisdom, and truth, and the beauty that exists in nature, rather than in artifice and concealment?

Every mother, from time to time, wonders about such things. You question whether you have any right to spend precious time—time that you could be spending in the company of the most important person in the entire world—getting highlights put into your hair, or having your nails painted a color you like. But you also wonder whether you have any right to pick up the cereal you want when there's a cereal that your child might like better. You wonder whether it's okay for you to buy the shirt that would make you feel confident at your presentation tomorrow rather than another toy car. You wonder whether it makes you a bad parent to not just want a Date Night—a night off from the responsibilities and worries and must-dos and should-nots that come along with parenting—but to really, deep down *need* one.

Does the choice to consider yourself mean that you are choosing not to consider your child?

In this chapter, I've written about quick pre-birth beauty routines to give you a little extra lift as you head toward a huge—and emotionally tumultuous—undertaking. I've told you to get eyelash extensions, because they're fun and weirdly practical if you're someone who enjoys having long eyelashes and is about to have a baby (and discover just how little time you have to apply actual mascara). I've recommended stretch mark solutions and skin-soothing masks and contouring techniques. And underneath it all, what I want you to understand is this:

It's not about makeup. It wasn't about makeup when I was standing under those bathroom lights and putting on lipstick before my subway ride home, and it wasn't about makeup when I put on some blush before getting in a taxicab and driving not just to the hospital, but toward my future. It's about finding a way to say to yourself, "I have fallen head over heels for my child, but that doesn't mean I can't love myself, too."

Pregnancy can be so hard. Motherhood can be so hard. There are physical challenges, of course—the cramps in your legs, the spots on your skin, the weight gain and stretch marks and places on your body that will honestly never return to what (and where) they once were—but even more, there is the sense that it's no longer about you. And that's true. From the moment your child arrives on the planet, he or she simply takes precedence; that's the way it is and the way it should be. Your own aches and exhaustion and worries get moved aside when your child is crying in the next room.

When your baby is born, you will think that she is so beautiful, and so special, and so deserving of all things wonderful: the freshest food, the cleanest air, the opportunity to go outside and just run and run and run. All of a sudden you'll see how simple life can be, and she'll remind you of all that easy joy in the world that you've spent years relegating to the place of myth. She'll want, and she'll need, and in turn, you'll want and need her to have not just those essentials that she *must* have (the food, the water, the bed), but those things that simply bring her joy (the stuffed puppy, the soft blanket, the cold washcloth on the hot day), and you'll want those things for her for no greater reason other than that she exists. She is a living person on this planet, and she deserves the opportunity to explore the greatest—and simplest—of joys.

You know who else is a living person on this planet?

You.

And you matter. As a parent, as someone's child yourself, and simply *because*. And the ways in which you can show yourself that you matter extend from your career goals to the attention you pay to your health to the tiny things you add to each day to make yourself feel beautiful; happy; like yourself.

I took very good care of myself when I was pregnant with my son. Better care of myself than I'd ever taken before—I always was a little thoughtless about my health—and I discovered that when I finally took the time to pay attention to my body and to what it wanted and needed, I felt *good*. And then I gave birth, and the vitamins ran out and never got replaced. I started eating whatever leftovers I had in the refrigerator instead of fresh fruit and vegetables, not exercising because I had trouble finding the time, sleeping too little and worrying too much and taking pills to help me sleep through my anxiety rather than actually *dealing* with it.

I looked forward to getting pregnant again because I was excited about having another baby, of course, but also because I looked forward to how good I knew I'd feel, because of how well I'd learned I take care of myself when it isn't really about me at all. But that's not the way it should be. Because while being gentle and thoughtful about your body when you're expecting a baby is so important (of course it is) it's not just "while you're pregnant" that you should be caring for yourself. It's before, and afterward, and all of the time.

The best part is, it's not a competition, a decision to allocate all that care to yourself or to your child. It's synergy. Your child's life is a beautiful, wonderful thing, and being completely absorbed in it isn't a danger; it's a privilege and an inevitability. It also doesn't need to pull every iota of focus away from your own weird, wonderful life. Because when you are good to yourself—when you're rested and when you're healthy, but also when you're following your dreams, taking time to do the things you love, and pursuing the meaning that defines who you are—you are not only a more relaxed, happy, and thoughtful parent . . . you are showing your child that self-care is not just a side note, but an imperative. You want your baby to learn to work hard, of course, but you also want him to remember that between all the work there is life, and whatever things help you to access those moments that make you feel most alive are things worth finding.

It's worth taking the time to care for the skin that you're in, baby.

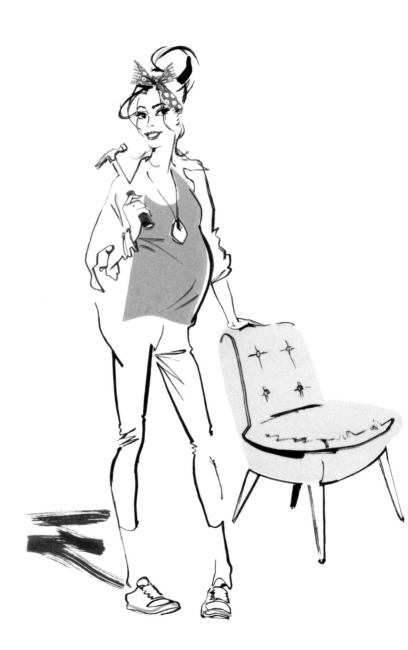

4

Decor & DIY

(PLEASE MAKE SURE YOU HAVE A PRENUP BEFORE YOU GO TO IKEA)

The Ikea Rocking Moose
(AND OTHER LESS-GOOD THINGS)

HERE IS A GOOD THING about Ikea: they have a really cute rocking moose that costs much, much less than the Restoration Hardware Rocking Lamb. Here is another good thing about Ikea:

. . .

. . .

Oh, wait. That's it.

I do love Ikea furniture, and I especially love their baby/toddler offerings, but I do not love *going* to Ikea. Not even a little bit, and especially not with my husband, who is generally a very kind, sweet man whom I love very much but who, somewhere between the Namjibs and Sklorens, becomes a person whom I despise with an all-consuming rage, whose every opinion I must disregard immediately upon issuance from his mouth, and who can do very literally nothing—I mean *nothing at all*—right.

I, in turn, become a shrieking harpy with a total inability to transcribe sixty-eight-digit numerical codes in a timely and accurate manner and a punishing desire to make my husband carry ALL OF THE PLANTS all the way through the Marketplace to the checkout while I decide which one I actually want to buy. (Allegedly.)

The first time we went to Ikea, Kendrick and I hated each other so much upon departure that we began to seriously question the very fabric of our relationship. If we couldn't make a simple purchase like a futon without a catastrophic breakdown in communication, wasn't it possible that we should just call this whole "marriage" thing off?

And then we got in the car and drove away, and realized: oh. We don't hate each other. We hate *the store*.

But Ikea is a necessary evil because 1) cheap; and 2) cute, and so I still think that you should go. Except I would like to clarify that I think you should go *right now*, while you're still pregnant and have not yet moved that thing that will make Ikea trips much, much worse in the future to the *outside* side of your body. Because let me tell you: as mind-bendingly bad as a trip to this place is when you are with your partner, it is worse when you are with your child.

After my husband and I moved our toddler and our dogs out of our one-bedroom New York City apartment into our first actual house (the kind with stairways and rooms that have things like doors), we all of a sudden found ourselves with space for items such as miniature circus tents and coat racks shaped like owls.

So we buckled our one-year-old into the car seat, plied him with as many snacks as the diaper bag could hold, and drove to the Ikea located just off of the Garden State Parkway in New Jersey. Not a spot that's especially exciting on the average day, but today? Today we were about to bring the party to Paramus, in the form of a child who would absolutely have to touch Every. Single. Item. in the store, and who would also very, very much need to be wayyy over there, behind or under that very large piece of furniture and completely hidden from sight, as opposed to in anything resembling close proximity to his loving mother and father.

Hold hands? I don't think so.

How this all ended: our son, having been prevented from making the store rounds all on his lonesome and just meeting us over at the checkout counter when he was done, morphed into a screaming extra from *Piranha 3-D*, complete with a full-body transformation into a completely rigid (but loud) plank of wood.

Mission: aborted. Home we go.

On subsequent trips, we made the following discoveries:

- Ikea is not open on Sundays (aka one of the two days out of the week when you have a shot in hell of convincing friends and relatives who have things like jobs to come help you wedge boxes the approximate size and weight of Subaru Outbacks into your Subaru Outback).

- When Ikea specifies that a bed comes in two packages, they sometimes forget to mention that the part of the bed that transforms it from a wooden hole into something that you can actually lie on (aka the slats) is sold in a separate, third package, for no especially good reason that I can discern other than to make me want to die.

- Everything in Ikea looks like a toy. Especially the things made of glass that my son wants to pick up and carry with him like a Snuggie.

- Ikea parking lots are really, really big and really, really hard to navigate, especially when you leave the juice box in your car by accident.

- Actually, everything having to do with Ikea is really, really big. Except they don't mention that until you reach the warehouse and see all the really, really big boxes and think about giving up, except you already hate your spouse and need to just buy the thing that you came to buy *right now* so that you never, ever have to come back to the store ever and can just leave already. Except you *can't* leave, because the goddamn box is too goddamn big. Goddamn it.

Don't even get me started on putting the crap that they sell together; I don't understand how any relationship sustains that level of stress.

HOW-TO: GO TO IKEA WITHOUT GETTING DIVORCED

It can be done. Or at least, you know: we're not divorced, so.

Eat: The cafeteria is there for a reason, and the reason is: meatballs. Eat them before you start your trip through the maze, and then eat them again before you confront the hell on earth for your wallet that is the Marketplace. They're not good, but they somehow make everything better.

Focus: Do not go to Ikea "just to take a look around." The end result of this decision will be you crying. Go with a goal, having done a pre-trip search on Ikea.com to decide exactly what you want (and the color you want it in), and when you get there go to the spot where they sell the thing you need, and get it, and then get out. No peeking at the glassware "just for a second." Definitely stay away from the pillows. And if you see a poster with a faux Warhol print on it, run. Remember: tears are always just moments away.

Keep in mind that size matters: Okay, so I get it: the point of Ikea is that it is cheap, and the reason that it is cheap is that nobody helps you. With anything. And this is okay if you are buying, say, a pot holder, and less okay if you are buying a wardrobe three times as tall as you are. If objects the size of your person or larger are on the menu, I am a firm believer in the power of Paying the Store to Do It. Pay the store to deliver it, and then pay the store to assemble it. It will still cost you less than buying a comparable item from a fancier store, and you will maintain your sanity (I value my own at approximately twenty dollars per hour; you'll have to make your own calculations on that point).

Reward thyself: Once you have made it through the madness that is the checkout line, take a second to discover the wonder that is the Ikea Kanelsnäcka (for those who do not speak Ikea: it's a cinnamon roll). You deserve it. You probably deserve six.

One of Life's Great Questions: Solved

You know, I've always wondered, if I suddenly discovered a strange man in my apartment, how would I react?

Last night, I got my answer.

Whenever I've imagined myself dealing with something like an intruder (and I do imagine such things), the scene unravels in a manner very similar to my SuperJordan car-crash scenario (see: Chapter 1, page 18): I notice a man (or hear a noise). My brain clicks immediately into high speed, generating numerous awe-inspiring escape scenarios. I calmly and constructively evaluate my surroundings and determine what, if anything, can be used for a weapon. And then I either brilliantly and stealthily escape without drawing notice, a grateful and loving dog tucked under each arm, or take a golf club to the intruder and emerge victorious. The fantasy is predominantly inspired by Ashley Judd (and Ashley Judd's character in *Kiss the Girls*, specifically), and generally ends with me getting a medal of some sort while wearing a really killer skirt suit.

It turns out that what I *actually* do is nothing at all except for scream like someone is charging at me full-tilt brandishing an ax.

Last night around 1:00 a.m. I was sitting at our dining table Googling baby names (really, there are few things more fun to Google in the world), and Kendrick was just getting back from walking the dogs. He was in the kitchen getting started on a few dishes, when out of the corner of my eye I noticed that there was most definitely someone else in our apartment. I turned, saw a man in a blue shirt walking slowly through our living room toward our bedroom, his back to me . . . and I began screaming. Five-alarm, Jamie Lee Curtis–in–*Halloween*–style screaming.

Or, according to my husband, screaming like I'd seen a cockroach, except at an even more higher-than-usual pitch that I attribute to the fact that I am about three seconds pregnant and thus even more prone than usual to slight mind losses of the shrieking variety. In any case, I apparently do this hysteria-for-no-especially-good-reason thing more than I realize, because Kendrick's response was not to jump into action wielding a samurai sword, but rather to ignore me completely and keep washing dishes.

By the time he realized that I was actually, legitimately frightened for actual, legitimate reasons, the poor guy standing in the center of our living room—who, as it turned out, was our extremely drunk neighbor, who had accidentally wandered into our place thinking it was his own—had been scared witless by the noise coming from the dining room (me) and had wandered back out in search of a less upsetting environment in which to continue being extremely drunk.

I would like to make special mention of our darling puppies here, because last night they really showed their mettle. When a man silently crept into our apartment, you know what Lucy and Virgil, tiny heroes, did? It can best be described using the words "radio silence." These dogs lose their goddamn minds over a squeak in the bathroom pipe and treat the poor FedEx guy like he's Cruella De Vil . . . but when it comes to an actual, for-real threat? Let's just go ahead and give that total stranger who has come into our home unbidden a nice tail wag. Maybe a lick.

But a bark? A growl? *Any indication whatsoever to our loving owners who feed us, house us, bathe us, and give us treats that there is a potential crisis in the making?*

Nah.

So that was exciting. And at least I've solved the question of how I respond to an intruder in my place.

Poorly.

Let the Sun Shine

. . . .

THE FIRST APARTMENT that my husband and I lived in after we got married was in Hell's Kitchen, a part of New York City that used to be extremely scary when I was growing up there in the '80s, and is now, just like the rest of Manhattan, extremely expensive. For the bargain price of slightly over $2,000 a month, we secured ourselves a third-floor walk-up apartment with a single bedroom almost exactly the size of our bed. The apartment had windows, which was better than the alternative, I suppose, but those windows also had a view of the brick wall of the building across the street, complete with a direct sightline into the living room of a large, large man who sometimes wandered around buck naked (yes, we had our very own Ugly Naked Guy). So we put up blinds. And curtains. And that meant that our already dark and "cozy" space became infinitely darker and "cozier."

Our next apartment, a fourth-floor walkup on New York City's Upper East Side (the Irish bars part, not the fancy part), had big kitchen windows and a more appetizing view, but it was also a railroad-style apartment (with the rooms arranged in a straight line), which meant that most of the place was completely sunshine-free. And the room that we chose for the nursery once we found out that we were expecting (for the carefully considered reason that it was our only option) was the very innermost room; it had no natural light whatsoever, and was illuminated by a single bare bulb way up in the center of our very high ceiling.

It was kind of depressing.

The thing is, you always want a home that feels warm and light, right? But when you have a baby it becomes especially important to create a living space that's peaceful, cozy, and just plain nice to exist in. Because guess what? You're about to spend a *lot* of time in it.

(Also, I blame Pinterest for making everyone I know, myself included, feel like in order to procreate they must also be capable of designing flawless, spectacularly adorable nurseries stocked with the full contents of the Pottery Barn Kids catalog and a whole bunch of perfectly executed DIY projects that would, in reality, require approximately $10,000 and probably a contractor and/or an architect. But that's another story.)

HOW-TO: BRIGHTEN UP YOUR LIVING SPACE

Transforming a dim, dreary room into a light and airy spot that you love to be in is not only totally possible, it's totally affordable. Small touches make a big difference when it comes to adding a bit of brightness.

Hang out: Try hanging a pretty fixture in the center of the room (ideally one with multiple bulbs) and additional smaller lights around the periphery. The goal is to create a wash of warm, beautiful light and to eliminate any dark, shadowy spots.

Wash of white: Keep the walls light; and try to incorporate light-reflecting fabrics (like all-white bedding) wherever possible.

Metallic moment: Consider adding some light-colored, patterned metallic wallpaper to a single wall (preferably the one opposite the door): the metallic detail will reflect the light and make the room feel larger while adding texture for warmth and interest.

Stay fresh: Install a ceiling fan to keep the air moving, or go for a cool retro version that sits on the floor.

Keep it natural: Choose "green" room scents (cucumber, grass, airy florals) rather than musky ones.

Stay on time: If you'd like a natural-light-free room to feel like it's keeping time with the world outside, consider hooking up a lamp with a dimmer option to a timer.

Keep it clean: Zero clutter will work wonders when it comes to making your space feel airy and inviting.

Go for greenery: Bring in some beautiful plants, but be sure to choose varieties that can live in the absence of natural light (African violets and snake plants do particularly well in dark areas). Or, if you're a professional plant-killer like me, pick up some gorgeous faux versions (or succulents, which are more or less unkillable).

PICK YOUR (FAUX) PLANT WISELY

Alas, price often really does make a difference when it comes to faux florals—both flowers and trees. But they're worth the investment, because when you find truly beautiful ones, you'll hold on to them forever. When buying faux plants, look for . . .

IMPERFECTIONS: Leaves and trunks with flaws and natural-textured petals that vary in color look much more real than their too-perfect cousins.

DETAILED STEMS: Little knobs, leaves, and irregularities make plants and flowers look like they came straight out of the garden. Also look for stems that have wire in them (so that you can twist them as you like) and are different lengths.

NATURAL-LOOKING BEDS: If the filler in the pot looks fake or boring, try covering it with some river rocks or gravel.

BOLD POTS: Rather than the plain black one that the plant came in, swap in a gorgeous ceramic or stone urn in a color that suits your decor.

Just Breathe

· · · · · · · · · · ·

BEFORE I HAD MY SON, I seriously did not get the obsession that people have with baby-head smell. I mean, didn't babies smell like . . . well, kind of like . . . poop? With gentle notes of vomit, perhaps?

Except then I had a baby, and: oh. *That* smell. I get it. These days I spend as much time as possible with my face planted in my son's scalp, basically trying to eat his hair while he's still young enough to be willing to actually let me do this.

Baby heads, as it turns out, smell like crack. Or like the olfactory equivalent of crack (which I gather doesn't actually smell very good). But they don't *always* smell good. And sometimes you want your house to smell good even when its inhabitants don't.

HOW-TO: YOUR HANDY ROOM-BY-ROOM SCENTING GUIDE

I'm sort of a nut about home scenting. I just think it's such a beautiful way to welcome people into your place while expressing a little bit of your personality. And really, there's nothing nicer than walking into a house that smells great. (Except for walking into a house that smells great because there are chocolate chip cookies in the oven, so if all else fails: do that.)

> **Entryway:** Go for florals, which provide a smooth transition from outside to inside. Except in New York City, where basically any scent you want to welcome guests into your home with will probably be preferable to the natural aroma of old Chinese food and car exhaust.

> **Living room:** Spicy scents and citruses heighten energy and get people feeling chatty. This is also a great place to play with seasonal scents. (Pumpkin pie! Pine needles!)

Kitchen: Citruses and herbal scents work well, but anything sharp and clean (like lemon verbena) will help eliminate cooking odors.

Bathroom: Because this is such a small area (and presumably one you and your guests don't spend all that much time in), it's a great place to try out something dramatic. Weird, even. Chocolate Mojito Sandalcarrot or whatever.

Bedroom: This is where you can get all romantic with lavender and tuberose, or create a cozy atmosphere with calming, mossy scents. You can also try using a sheet spray that compliments the scent you've chosen for the room (for example, a sage candle blends nicely with lavender water spritzed onto pillows before bedtime).

God, Baby Furniture Is Expensive

· · · · · · · · · · ·

BEFORE I GOT ANCIENT AND BORING and started being far more interested in how large and comfortable my couch is than pretty much anything else in the world, I hated buying furniture. It ranked wayyy down there on the list of Things I Am Looking Forward To Doing Today (Or Ever) along with buying running shoes.

I like furniture-shopping *now*—the sales floor at Crate & Barrel is one of my favorite places to spend a Saturday afternoon—but for years and years I hated even the idea of it, mostly because things like coffee tables and armchairs are often unfathomably expensive, and besides: why would you buy furniture, I reasoned, when there was so much of it sitting right there on the street, all free and stuff?

In New York City, you see—and especially in neighborhoods that tend to attract lots of transient youths who switch boyfriends and roommates every year or so, resulting in a semiannual hop from one walk-up apartment to another—weekend mornings are basically street-furniture bonanzas. When my husband and I lived on the Upper East Side (on a block especially laden with twentysomethings who were constantly moving in and out), only about one third of the furniture in our place was actually ours. The love seat in the "office" (aka the hallway aka the future nursery) was formerly our downstairs neighbor's; the kitchen hutch, table, and chairs had been abandoned by the apartment's previous renters; the living room couch was a hand-me-down from my parents; and the floor lamp, side table, desk chair, strange metal flower wall hanging, and china cabinet adorned with fish drawn by a respectably famous graffiti artist?

Found them on the street. Dragged them upstairs. (Or rather, made my husband drag them upstairs.)

Now, hold on, because I can hear you screaming "BEDBUGS" at me from all the way over here.

True. Bedbugs were a bit of a problem in NYC for a while there, and that combined with an extreme bug phobia contributed to me placing a hold on the straight-from-the-streets finds. But I still love hunting for furniture at yard sales, flea markets, and thrift stores, and think these places can be total meccas when it comes to decorating your home, provided you exercise a wee bit of caution.

Get Thee to (Furniture) Rehab

. . . .

ONE OF THE MAJOR REASONS I love working with hand-me-down (or found) furniture is that there's no pressure—you can go way over-the-top with color and pattern, and the worst thing that can happen is that you have to get rid of something that didn't exactly break the bank in the first place. Of course we don't *want* to be trashing all our hard work, though, so when it comes to the rehabbing proceed as carefully as you would if you'd paid a fortune for the piece (also worth mentioning: when you're working with used furniture, a slapdash approach is even more apparent).

WOOD REFINISHING BASICS

Before painting or staining a wooden piece, you might want to restore the wood; I tend not to do this too often because I'm impatient, but also because it just isn't a big deal to have a chip or uneven spot here and there. But if you want to give the wood a little fixing-up, here's what you do:

1. Strip off the old paint or sand off the old stain (start with 80 grit and move up to 150 grit or 220 grit, using a tack cloth to remove sawdust between sandings).

2. Sand again to smooth down the wood. Wipe away dust with a clean rag.

3. Fill in any damaged areas or cracks with wood putty and let dry.

4. Sand down again to create a smooth surface.

FURNITURE PAINTING BASICS

Painting furniture can be a little time-consuming, but it's also fairly unscrewupable: just apply three thin coats of paint using a decent brush, and you're good.

1. Put down a (big) drop cloth, or lots and lots of newspaper.

2. Whenever possible, strip furniture that's already painted and sand it down along the grain of the wood.

3. Use water-based paint on wood furniture.

4. Gloss paint shows *everything*, so only use it if the surface you're painting is pristine (use semi-gloss or matte for a more forgiving finish).

5. Nail polish remover gets the stains off of furniture/floors that have been splattered, but you should spot-test first to ensure that you won't take off anything you don't want to.

WOOD DISTRESSING BASICS

If you find a piece that's respectably new-looking but would prefer a distressed finish, no worries: you can DIY that as well.

1. Sand the wood lightly along the grain, concentrating on the areas that would naturally get the most wear and tear (like armrests and corners).

2. Take a hammer and (lightly!) bang the sides of the piece, wherever denting would naturally occur.

3. Rub a few areas that you want to look extra-distressed with a wire brush or Brillo pad. You can even use an awl or chisel to make little holes in the wood, if you like.

4. If you'd like to try a stained look and don't feel like heading to the store, try pouring some strong coffee over the piece, and add more coats until you achieve the desired effect.

The Tale of the
Mushroom in the Night

. . . .

I GREW UP IN NEW YORK CITY. And in New York City, people do not own homes; they rent $3,000 per month shoeboxes that are "really close to a lot of great restaurants." Or maybe they own these boxes, because they have half a million dollars lying around and think that seven hundred square feet is a good thing to spend that half a million dollars on.

Or maybe they own both boxes in the city and actual houses in places like the Hamptons. I don't personally know people like this (although I did in high school, because I went to a very fancy Upper East Side school with lots of very fancy people), but maybe you do. I'm sure you guys have a lot of fun splashing around in gorgeous swimming pools in your Calypso caftans all summer long. Congratulations on winning at everything.

My point is that home ownership in New York City is not really the norm—and especially not when you're still within spitting distance of your college years. When I moved back to the city after a few years in Los Angeles, I knew that as long as I lived within the confines of the five boroughs I'd almost certainly be a shoebox-renter. That was fine by me for the time being, because I was twenty-seven and newly married and busy enjoying the many things the city has to offer to offset the truly unconscionable housing situation . . . but I also knew that I had a major soft spot for actual houses with things like actual yards.

Barbecues. Blow-up pools sitting in the grass. Bedroom doors. Closets. You know.

Being really close to a lot of great restaurants is nice, but I'd rather have a kitchen with a stove that you do not have to light with a match while lying on your back on the floor, and that does not have a 40 percent chance of shooting a ball of fire into your face each and every time you do this. (Oh, I didn't mention? The stove in our last apartment tried to kill me.) And perhaps some semblance of peace, as opposed to wasted frat guys spilling out of clubs called Halo or Aubergine at four in the morning all DUUUDE TEXT HER RIGHT NOWWW.

I'm old, what can I say? I don't care about your texting drama, and at four in the morning I care so much less, I can't even tell you.

In other words: I always knew that one day I'd want to pack up and head to more spacious pastures. And when we found out we were expecting our son seemed as good of a time to get that show on the road as any.

I had this very idyllic, very sunbeams-and-sparkles picture in my head of what living in a house would be like. And when we eventually found and moved into our house it was very much like I'd pictured: idyllic, sunbeams and sparkles, et cetera et cetera. I even had a hammock. It was paradise.

And then I found the mushroom.

Before we go any further, I need to explain something to you: one of the major problems with writing a book as opposed to inviting each and every human being reading these words over to my house so I can just tell you these stories in person is that I cannot take you by the hand and walk you from room to room, showing you that I am a non-hoarder-type individual who lives in a completely habitable abode with things like cleaning products that get used on a regular basis.

I'm not obsessive (although my husband, who is the kind of man who thinks that the coffee table is as good of a spot as any to put his dirty socks, would probably beg to differ on this point), but I am pretty neat. The mail is piled up and ignored, yes, but it's piled up and ignored *in the right spot*; the disaster zone created by my son's toys has been corralled in the playroom, and the tops of picture frames get dusted . . . well, not "frequently," necessarily, but certainly frequently enough that you would not be horrified.

I'm not completely gross. I promise.

The reason that I'm belaboring this point: because when what I'm about to tell you about happened, I got worried that I might be. Gross.

A few months after we moved in I was giving my son a bath, and since our house doesn't have a bathtub other than the one in the basement (aka the room where Monster Spiders live and I do not go), what "giving my son a bath" means is putting him in a large plastic tub on the floor of our upstairs bathroom along with a bunch of toy boats. Now, kids like to splash a lot, but I figure, what, am I going to deprive my son of this essential childhood joy? No, I'm going to just wipe up the water after the bath is done and he's in bed.

Bath was done, child was in bed, and I went to wipe up the water. And sitting there, right at the edge of my shower . . .

Was a mushroom.

Not a little teeny-tiny thing that I could just run over with a paper towel and be like, "nope, didn't see that, not even a little bit." We're talking a two-inch tall *plant*.

(Just so you're aware, even writing these words is so horrifying to me that I'm basically in a puddle right now. But let's soldier on.)

The next thing that I did was panic, obviously, because: mushroom. (Here is the point where I'm going to make sure that you know something that I did not know at the time, but certainly do now: whatever you do, do not Google "mushroom growing in bathroom." You will be sorry, and then you will not sleep or eat ever again in your life.)

My mother, incidentally, does not understand why this was such a hugely distressing discovery. Nor does my husband, so apparently not everyone has this kind of a reaction to the presence of small trees growing out of their floors. While I don't understand that at all—how is a mushroom in your shower not an automatic Thing That a Rational Person Cannot Handle?— if you're having a similarly tough time understanding why I freaked out quite as much as I did, try this: you know how some people feel about the word "moist"? How it just makes them shudder uncontrollably from some primal part of their soul?

That's how I feel about the words "there is a mushroom in your shower."

They make me want to faint.

So after I worked on not-fainting for a while, I called my contractor, who was the first responsible homeowner-type person whose name popped into my head (and who I'm sure was thrilled to get a late-night ring from the young lady whose floors he had worked on a few months earlier). He very nicely explained to me that while discovering members of the fungi family coming through the floor of your bathroom is odd (and, yes, gross), it is also something that does tend to happen when you have a lot of water dripping onto the same spot on your tiles for an extended period of time (ahem), especially if one of those tiles is loose-ish (oops). The next thing that he said was that I should rip up my floors and take a look at what was underneath.

Now, obviously I went ahead and paid someone to do that. Not because I am a billionaire with nothing better to do than throw cash at people, but rather because while I am actually quite good at dealing with about 99 percent of the issues that home ownership tosses my way, salad fixings sprouting from my tiles falls firmly into the category of I Will Pay You Whatever You Want Me To Pay You So That I Do Not Have To Deal With This.*

---

*For those of you on the edges of your seats, it turned out fine. The "problem" was confined to about two square inches of space that were bleached to the point of near-disintegration and then covered back up. This was also done by someone other than me. Obviously.

More dramatic home ownership moments over the past couple of years:

- An incident in the living room where I slipped on the inexplicably soaking-wet floor, only to look up and discover oh, hello: that's the upstairs shower, coming in through the ceiling;

- An incident in the backyard involving a turtle (there was a *turtle*—in our *backyard*) that ended with me crying because we could not keep him;

- A second incident in the backyard involving a baby blue jay that also ended with me crying because we could not keep him. (What can I say? The closest thing to tiny, forlorn abandoned animals that you find when you grow up in New York City are teeny baby cockroaches, or maybe—if you're lucky—teeny baby rats);

- An incident involving me alone in my house one night accompanied only by a creature called a "spricket," which, for those of you who do not live in places where these little guys prosper, is more or less a cross between a spider and a cricket, and comes only in XL size. Basically, it's a tarantula whose primary defense mechanism is to jump. *At you.* It is a spider-cricket . . . that attacks. And I have them *in my house.*

Also, did you know that water pipes in hundred-year-old houses have a tendency to turn into ice flues when it is cold out? They do.

So know this: if you buy a house, you may very well have to contend with things like sprouting floorboards, living room waterfalls, ice pipes, and zombie tarantula-crickets. Or maybe you won't have to deal with those specific things . . . but there will be something.

There's always something.

Which isn't to say that home ownership isn't wonderful. It is. I just need you to be prepared. And own bleach.

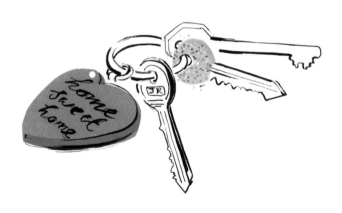

Random Acts of Responsibility

. . . .

KIDS ARE WONDERFUL. They are magical little creatures whose mere existence in your life will make it better in nearly every way possible. It's true.

Something else that's true: kids come with a lot of paperwork. Vaccination records, 529 accounts, day-care applications, et cetera et cetera and on into eternity (or at least until they graduate from college, at which point you can do what my mother did, which is hand them an enormous file full of their documents and say "This is your problem now"). And while these kinds of documents are always pretty important to keep track of, they're *especially* important when they have to do with your kids, because nothing will make you feel like a terrible parent faster than realizing that not only do you not know your child's social security number . . . you don't know where you might begin even *looking* for it.*

I know: filing sounds boring. Reading about filing sounds worse. But bear with me, because I promise: putting ten minutes into filing each week will save you on both time and gray hairs later, when you discover that you really, really, really need that pediatrician's letter/Buy Buy Baby receipt/breast-feeding pump manual and poof, there it is, right there in that

---

*I just realized, while writing these words, that I do not know my child's social security number. But do I know the location of the file where I will be able to find it? I do. BOOM.

little folder that you so wisely allocated to it.

As a bonus: every so often, my husband will be like, "Hey honey? Do you have that random piece of paper that I handed you eight months ago without telling you what it was or what I wanted you to do with it?" And in response, I get to say, "Why, yes, dear. It's filed right here in an appropriately titled, easy-to-access folder. May I get you a photocopy?"

And then I win for the day. So I think you should try it.

HOW-TO: OLD-SCHOOL (AND AWESOME) FILING SYSTEM

Sure, you can scan all your important papers and file them in folders on your computer. That would be really smart, and would save a ton of space. I am self-aware enough to know that I would never do this in a million years. I'd say to myself that I would, and then the first time I was presented with a scan-requiring occasion what would happen to that paper is that it would go into a pile, where it would sit awaiting my decision to actually deal with it, and I'd never deal with it, and then it would get lost.

For some things—like filing—going old-school just makes life easier.

- At the start of a new year, open up a new Redweld folder (one of those huge reddish accordion-style folders) and write the year clearly on the front. Then use smaller file folders to create subcategories (e.g. "Cars," "Utilities," "Manuals," "Retirement Accounts," et cetera).

• Keep a basket (basically an "Inbox") in a convenient spot and throw everything that will eventually need to be dealt with into the basket. Once a week (or once a month), sit down and go through the basket and organize everything into folders. This lets you be lazy on a day-to-day basis and only have to actually file once in a while, while ensuring that you don't lose any important documentation.

That's it. It's old-school and it works and I love it.

STAY ORGANIZED

- Keep the present year's file and last year's file easily accessible; all other years can be (neatly) stored away.

- Don't be afraid to open up a new folder even if you only have one or two things to go in it; it's much better to have clear labels for everything than to end up with a million random things stuffed into the back of your file because you have no idea where else to put them.

- That said, there will occasionally be papers that you aren't sure what to do with. I keep a "Random Stuff" folder for these papers, and just try not to be too liberal with what goes in there.

- Important original documents that you'll need to access repeatedly over time (for example, social security documents and marriage certificates) should be kept in a separate file folder labeled "Important Household Documents" that you move into the present year's file every January or keep in their own Redweld (in a very safe place). You'll always know where they are, and you'll never have to go digging around in your attic for something you absolutely need right this very second.

- Very important personal documents present an exception to my preference for old-school methods; you should keep the originals in a file, but should also have scanned copies backed up on your computer just in case.

TO PET OR NOT TO PET

I have been in an argument with my dogs pretty much since the day we found out we were expecting our first child.

What's that, you ask? "How can one argue with a dog?" Let's take a quick look at the situation here.

Lucy, my sweet-as-pie eight-pound shih tzu who does not move during sunlight hours, and who is so stationary during the portion of the day traditionally dedicated to activity that she must be carried into the backyard to be reminded to pee, transforms into Speedy Gonzales between the hours of 1:00 a.m. and 5:00 a.m. If she is on the bed, she must be down (and must have my assistance in order to get there). If she is off the bed, she must be on it (and, again: must be physically assisted in this pursuit). She must sleep on my face. Then she must lick it. Maybe scratch it. She is so thirsty that she must drink All of the Water, and then let me know that more is required. And at some point, usually when I am about to cry because I am so tired, she must go downstairs and bark. At the wall. For the sole apparent purpose of waking up my kid.

Virgil, my twenty-pound Lhasa apso, is such an asshole I cannot even tell you. He's sort of like a very cute hurricane, and responds to our efforts to get him to do anything other than panic (about everything) as if we are trying to explain quantum physics. Reason, negative feedback, positive feedback, and an endless array of evidence that no matter what he does, he will never be permitted to live the madcap life of nonstop foot-licking, couch-top wind-sprints, and in-house excretion that he dreams of? All of these have next-to-no impact in the face of his overwhelming need to freak the F out. About everything.

As an example: Virgil is absolutely convinced that our mailman is trying to murder him. I am certain of this because our mailman has come to the door approximately six hundred times since we moved into our new house, and each of these six hundred times Virgil has tried to attack him (and been yelled at). And still: every single day at noon, when the mailman steps onto our front porch, Virgil forgets that history has shown him (over and over) that the door will remain closed even if he hurtles himself into it (over and over) with neck-breaking force. The door will remain intact, the mailman will deposit the mail, and the little mail van will putter back to life and drive away down the street. This will happen every single day like clockwork, no matter how much panic and noise is associated with the process. And yet something about the mailman's appearance causes unrest in my dog that is so deeply rooted, so profound, that he simply must not give up.

This time, he says to himself, *this time I will put an end to it*.

Another example: because Virgil could not restrain himself from launching off of the wall surrounding our backyard into the thicket of fur-ensnaring branches below (over and over), I spent a small fortune building a high fence around our property.

Because despite the fact that he is an asshole, I love him and I want him to not die. And then he found the one spot that I failed to secure, and now uses it to escape and then catapult himself down our road toward the sole location in our town— the highway several hundred yards away—most likely to kill him. He does this every single time our back door opens, and especially does this when I have just gotten out of the shower and must thus run down a hill after him wearing only a robe.

Once, I spent three hours constructing an elaborate meal for myself and our son because I was four months pregnant and I wanted to do something nice and decadent, and a full afternoon of chopping, stirring, and sautéing ended with the two of us sitting down to a beautifully set table, super-hungry and super-excited to start in on this wonderful meal. It was at that exact moment that Virgil threw up, directly onto my feet. And then there was that time during my son's potty-training period when the toilet overflowed so dramatically that I went flying out of our bathroom screaming the word "SHITWATER," and Lucy recognized her one opportunity to eat all the poop she wanted unhindered by her erstwhile master. I believe my dog consumed an amount of fecal matter equivalent to half her body weight in the space of thirty seconds. It was actually a pretty amazing achievement.

The take-home from this is as follows: if you are expecting a child and also thinking about getting a dog, know that they will wake you up during the precious twenty seconds during which your child is sleeping peacefully, vomit on you when you are trying to have a nice dinner, and eat poop. They're also cute, and get really excited when you come back through the door after a five-second walk down the driveway to take out the garbage.

Do as you will.

HOW-TO: TRAIN YOUR DOGS TO BE NOT-ASSHOLES

I don't know. If you know, please write a book. I will read it.

Get It Done

· · · · · · · · · · ·

HISTORICALLY, I'D RATE myself around a seven on the Competency Scale. I know how to check my oil, but I don't know how to change a tire. I know how to fix a blown fuse, but not how to handle anything at all having to do with my remote control (history has proven that all I have to do to initiate a semi-permanent and total shutdown of every single feature of my television is to hit the fast-forward button while watching a DVR-ed show).

When we moved into our house, though, the degree to which I had to display a reasonable amount of can-do-ness in a wide range of situations suddenly went way, way up. Pipes frozen? Figure it out. Babysitter's car cemented into the snow-filled driveway? Figure it out. Dog refuses to stay in backyard and insists on leaping joyfully into the tick-and-bramble-filled woods that surround the house every single time the door is opened? Figure it out (or tell the dog good luck, have a blast, and keep the groomer on speed-dial).

Let me tell you: I thought that I would hate all this figuring-it-out, that it would be exhausting and difficult and time-consuming. It is all those things. It's also remarkable and often-times astonishingly exciting, simply because there is nothing like the feeling of getting that pipe to unfreeze, or sensing that those tires suddenly found traction, or watching your dog crash into the fence that now separates him from the paradise beyond the backyard, and knowing: *I fixed it.*

A year after we moved, my husband was admitted to a full-time business school program located in another state. Very quickly, we realized that the commute that we had thought would be "a pain, but possible" was just totally crazy, and decided that the best course of action was to have him rent an apartment to spend weeknights in . . . for the next two years.

I wanted to be supportive, and brave, and unfailingly loving, and all those things that I am when I picture marital challenges playing out in my head, but what I actually was, was really, really scared. Because as much as I'd strengthened my ability to handle all the strange and unforeseeable and daunting tasks that come along with living in a house for which you are responsible, I still liked that I had someone taller than me hanging around when I needed to change a lightbulb. I liked that I could be responsible for taking out the trash, and know that someone else was going to take care of carrying out the boxes for recycling. It's nice, the knowledge that while sure, you *can* do everything on your own, you don't necessarily *have* to.

All of a sudden, I had to.

It was, as I'd feared, scary. And it was also one of the best things that ever happened to me.

The first night that Kendrick was gone, I ate dinner with our son and then set him down in front of *Sesame Street* while I went into the kitchen to clean up. I noticed it then, of course— the fact that it was just me loading the dishwasher, just me scrubbing the pots, just me wiping the sink, just me doing the things that Kendrick usually does either alongside me or on his own while I'm off doing other stuff. But then I looked down, and next to the garbage pail I saw a little fluff-thing.

I'm lazy about fluff-things. I rarely pick them up; I think they're vaguely creepy (there is always the chance that a bug is in there somewhere), and I also sort of assume that . . . I don't know . . . they'll disintegrate, or that someone else will deal with them.

But that night I looked at the fluff-thing sitting there next to the garbage can, and all of a sudden it hit me: if I did not pick it up, it would be there the next morning when I woke up. And then it'd be there the morning after that.

Nothing—not one single thing—would happen if I didn't make it so.

If I didn't let out the dogs, no one would hear them whine and open the door. If I didn't pick up the milk, no one would swing by the store on the way home. If I didn't kill that spricket, it would live in my house and have spricket babies that would terrorize me forever and ever.

One morning, I stepped out my back door and directly into a spider web the size of a hammock, presided over by a spider approximately the circumference of a walnut. And freaked the F out. And then dealt with it.

Leaks in the bathroom, dings in the car, trips to Costco, taking the garbage out, bringing the dogs in, changing the bulbs, fixing the dishwasher, making the food, giving the baths, trying to create at least moderately educational experiences for my child, and getting work done somewhere in between all of this. Small things like the fact that I don't like emptying the catch in the sink because it's slimy, and big things like the fact that our son hit his head one night and it bled and I wanted someone there next to me while I called the pediatrician and applied pressure with a paper towel. It's all ordinary stuff, of course, and it's stuff that I should be able to (and, for the most part, am able to) handle. But it also sometimes feels like a lot.

Because the last time I was doing everything myself, it was just "myself" I was doing it for. These days there are more of us, and there's more to do. And all those to-dos can be overwhelming from time to time, but they've also been teaching me to just do them, whatever "they" may be. Even if it's late. Even if I'm tired. Even if I don't want to: I've got to get it done, one way or another.

And so that night, standing there all alone in my kitchen, I picked up the fluff-thing. (With a paper towel. You know: just in case.)

And guess what? Fluff-things? They're just fluff. Mushrooms are just mushrooms. All the stuff that can seem so intimidating . . . when you look at it in the light of day, it's actually not so scary at all. It's just stuff you've got to do.

So you get it done.

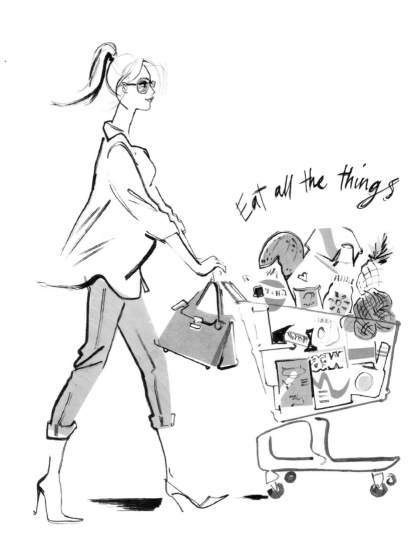

Eat all the things

5

Eating & Entertaining

(AND THE VERY WORST PARTY IN THE WORLD)

Eat All the Things

THERE IS THIS THING that you probably shouldn't do when you're pregnant. But I'm going to tell you to do it anyway, because there are lots of things that people say that you "shouldn't do" when you're pregnant, and many of them you truly should not do, but this one I think you actually should. It's so much fun.

Go to the grocery store when you're starving.

Now, going to the grocery store while hungry, for me, is always an exercise in bizarre purchasing choices, but when I'm pregnant? Oh my god, the amazing things I return home with. Last time I went, for example, I came home with three different varieties of pickles because I'm a walking stereotype (in my defense, bread and butter pickles are pretty much a whole separate food group from half-sour ones), two packages of celery because it looked so damn delicious (and we all know that if there is one thing that celery does not look, it is "delicious"), a four-pound brisket (with accompanying vegetables and/or starches? Of course not), and a box of chocolate-marshmallow pies that are made in the Little Debbie factory and that basically taste like cardboard-wrapped pillows, and I don't care. Ate them; loved them.

Eating is fun all of the time; we know this. But when you're pregnant? Funner.

Now, let's get one thing straight: I'm by no means advising you to treat your body like a garbage dump for the nine months of gestation. Obviously we should be getting our vegetables and our protein, and taking our prenatal vitamins, and drinking our water, but you know what I call a pregnancy without the occasional shot of Fluffernutter? A missed opportunity. Don't miss your opportunity.

My favorite thing about eating bizarre and/or excessively decadent things when pregnant: sure, people (the kinds of people who prefer kale to Nutella, who are the kinds of people I don't trust) will still tsk-tsk you about your nutritional choices . . . but really, everyone loves a pregnant lady with a milk shake. Everyone.

And the ones who don't will discover very quickly that

when it comes to pregnant women and cravings, a rational evaluation of nutritional content is not only somewhat besides the point, it is likely to make them mad.

And no one wants to make a pregnant lady mad. No one.

As an example, I posted a picture of my Best Sandwich in the World (see page 193) on Instagram once, and a healthy-living-type colleague of mine wrote something along the lines of, "Jordan, we really need to have a talk about what you put into your body. What you eat, the baby eats!"

Those are some fighting words, girlfriend.

But here's another fun thing about pregnancy: you don't have to even acknowledge or deal with statements like this; all you have to do is get a sort of wide-eyed look about you and gesture wildly at your stomach while saying "CHOCO-LATE," and most people will get out of your way and go back to their salads.

Also, try to eat salads when you're pregnant. I mean, I don't. But I feel like I should probably put that in here anyway.

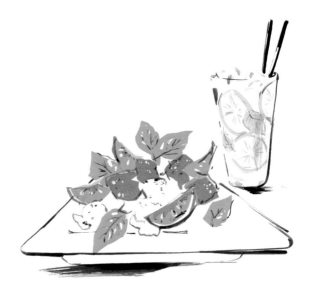

Things I Want to Eat

. . . .

WHEN I WAS PREGNANT WITH MY SON, I didn't actually have any "cravings," per se. Except for coffee, which I had never especially liked before but suddenly desired with the heat of a thousand suns. (The amount of restraint it took to limit myself to my doctor-approved one cup a day was second only to the amount of restraint it took for me to not land my best haymaker on the Starbucks barista who suggested that I "might like a decaf instead" when I ordered my morning joy.)

With my daughter, things are a little different. Sure, it's an old wives' tale, the "craving sweets means you're having a girl" thing, but the extent to which I was not especially a sweets person pre-second-pregnancy, and then suddenly absolutely required Häagen-Dazs Chocolate-Chocolate Chip ice cream if I was going to make it through the evening? To me, that said that there was something very different going on with Take Two.

In this chapter, we're not going to talk about things that you "should" eat, or things that make for anything resembling a balanced diet; there are plenty of books out there written by people who know much more about nutrition than I do (which is nothing). This is very literally a chapter about the things that I like eating when I am pregnant, and that I think that you might like eating, too. Why? Because it's my book, and one thing that I am a total expert on is the topic of Stuff That I Like To Eat. So here we go.

CUCUMBER YOGURT WITH MINT AND OLIVE OIL

This is less of a "recipe" than "a bunch of things I like all mixed together" . . . but that's okay, because it's so good. And fresh, and light, and perfect for breakfast or for a snack. Or for 3:00 a.m.

Serves 1

1 cup Greek yogurt

¼ cup English cucumber, diced

2 or 3 leaves of mint, finely chopped

Coarse sea salt, to taste

½ teaspoon olive oil

Pita bread

Just mix together the first three ingredients (adding salt to taste; I like quite a lot), then drizzle over the olive oil. Garnish with another mint leaf if you feel like making it look fancy or like putting it on Instagram.

Serve with a few pita triangles on the side.

PUMPKIN PIE OATMEAL

When I was pregnant with my first child and had time in the morning to eat things other than Eggo waffles, I went through a phase where I made awesome oatmeal-based concoctions nearly every single day. This one, which basically tastes like an autumn morning in a bowl, was my favorite by far.

Serves 1

1 cup milk (more or less, depending on how thick you like your oatmeal)

½ cup quick-cook rolled oats

¼ cup canned pumpkin puree

¼ teaspoon pumpkin pie spice

¼ teaspoon cinnamon

¼ teaspoon salt

½ banana, sliced

¼ cup walnuts, chopped

2 tablespoons maple syrup

Whipped cream (optional)

Bring the milk to a boil in a saucepan.

Add the oats, then stir in the pumpkin, spices, and salt. Cook, stirring constantly, about 2 minutes (or as indicated by the package directions on the rolled oats).

Pour the oatmeal into a bowl and add sliced banana, walnuts, maple syrup, and whipped cream (if desired).

CALIFORNIA SCRAMBLE

When I first moved to L.A., I briefly dated an actor who was all into healthy, California-type things like hiking and egg whites. He later ended up getting cast on a TV show playing a desert island castaway, so presumably his taste for rabbit food worked out in his favor. I do not enjoy rabbit food. But our favorite place to go for brunch, the Griddle, presented an excellent compromise: he would order sprouts, and I would order pancakes and a mimosa. Every once in a while, though, he'd order this one dish, and despite the fact that my pancakes were really pretty spectacular, I kept sneaking bites of his. Because yeah, it was healthy . . . but it was also very, very (very) good. This is it, basically.

Serves 2

1 tablespoon olive oil

½ onion, finely diced

4 large eggs (or sub in 6 egg whites
   if you want to go the extra mile)

Splash of milk

2 tablespoons butter

1 tomato, diced

½ cup fresh mozzarella, diced

¼ avocado, diced

Salt and pepper, to taste

In a frying pan, heat a tablespoon of the olive oil and sauté the onions in the oil until just translucent. Set aside.

Whisk together the eggs and milk in a small bowl.

Heat the butter in a frying pan until foaming, and then add the eggs, scrambling them constantly while they cook so they come out all nice and fluffy.

Toss in the onion, tomato, mozzarella, and avocado. Season with salt and pepper to taste.

BRINNER

What is brinner, you ask? Brinner is when you eat breakfast for dinner, and it is the best, most satisfying, wonderful meal in the world. Lest you think I'm exaggerating: I ate this a minimum of once per week throughout each of my pregnancies, and probably would have eaten it more often than that save for the fact that my husband appears to think that there are other meals that could be termed "the best, most satisfying, wonderful meal in the world" (he is wrong).

Another bonus: something about this dish (maybe the mix of "good" fats and carbs?) is both filling and stomach-settling, making it the perfect thing to eat when you're not feeling quite right (like, say, during that first trimester).

Serves 2

Olive oil

5 or 6 potatoes, diced
into ¼ -inch pieces

1 medium yellow onion,
diced

Generous sprinkling of garlic powder

Salt and pepper, to taste

1 ripe avocado, diced

4 large eggs

Splash of milk

In a large pan, heat the olive oil and then sauté the potatoes and onions with the garlic powder and salt and pepper to taste until tender, stirring more or less constantly. This is going to take a while—like 20 to 30 minutes—so you can parboil the potatoes and then just sauté them for the last few minutes if you like, but I find the process oddly meditative and relaxing. Plus, if you take the time to cook the potatoes and onions this way you'll end up with lots of burn-y bits to scrape off the bottom, which only adds to the flavor of the final product.

Remove the pan from the heat. Toss in the diced avocado, and add a little extra seasoning if you like.

Either fry the eggs or poach them, whichever you prefer.

Serve by plating a scoop or two of hash and setting an egg on top.

SLOW-COOKER DECONSTRUCTED VEGETABLE POT PIE

I cannot eat chicken when I am pregnant. It's my friend Morgan's fault: when she was pregnant she told me that she couldn't eat chicken, and the reason that she gave me (which I'm not going to repeat because it's too gross to put in a chapter about food) freaked me out so much that it resulted in me never, ever being able to eat chicken again while feeling anything less than completely 100 percent. For those of you looking for flavor and heartiness minus that ingredient, let me present: this.

Serves 4 to 6

1 medium yellow onion, diced

4 or 5 medium red potatoes, cut into ¼ -inch cubes

1 or 2 leeks (white and green parts only), thinly sliced

2 handfuls of baby carrots, chopped

1 small bag frozen peas (or use fresh ones)

1 ½ cups dried northern beans (navy beans are good, too)

1 teaspoon fresh thyme, chopped

¼ cup flour

4 cups vegetable broth

4 tablespoons butter, cut into 1 tablespoon pats

Salt and pepper, to taste

Throw the first seven ingredients into the slow cooker and mix lightly.

In a small bowl, whisk together the flour and vegetable broth, and then pour the mixture over the vegetables. Gently stir to combine.

Place the pats of butter on top of the vegetables. Cook on high for about three hours, then on low for another five or six hours. Season to taste.

Serve topped with homemade biscuits (see page 190).

FETTUCCINE WITH SWEET TOMATO SAUCE AND ASPARAGUS

I have a weird thing for Prego. I think it's because my mom used to use it as a base for pasta sauce when I was a little girl, just tossing in things like mushrooms and onions to jazz it up. I mean, I totally get it: you're supposed to like homemade sauce best, and yes, it's wonderful, but . . .

Goodness, is Prego delicious. It's sort of like McDonald's hamburgers versus one of those thirty-dollar ones with things like truffles and diamonds in them or whatever: they're just totally different categories of food, and wonderful in their own ways. I think, however, that what makes me like Prego is—rather unfortunately— the same thing that makes it a less-great option than homemade sauce: all that added sugar that's present in pretty much anything that you buy pre-made.

This pasta dish is fresh and light, and has that touch of sweetness that I'm looking for without actually being loaded up with sugar. I've been making this recipe for years, and have tweaked it to make it as straightforward and simple as possible. It takes about fifteen minutes start to finish, and is a major crowd-pleaser.

1 bunch asparagus

2 to 3 tablespoons olive oil

Salt, to taste

1 medium yellow onion, diced

2 teaspoons fresh garlic, minced

24-ounce can diced tomatoes

1 package fresh pasta of your choice

1 teaspoon balsamic vinegar

¾ cup fresh whole-milk ricotta

Pepper, to taste

Preheat the oven to 400°F.

Trim the tough ends (the lower third) from the asparagus and lightly drizzle with 1 tablespoon of olive oil and sea salt, then roast for 5 to 8 minutes (or until fork-tender).

In a heavy-bottomed saucepan, heat the remainder of the olive oil and cook the onion until just translucent, adding the garlic for the last minute or two of cooking and stirring constantly to prevent burning.

Add the tomatoes and turn down the heat. Let the sauce simmer for about 10 minutes.

Meanwhile, cook the pasta according to the package directions (fresh pasta should only take a couple of minutes).

Stir the balsamic vinegar and ricotta into the sauce, and season with salt and pepper to taste.

Just before serving, cut the roasted asparagus into 1-inch pieces and toss it with the pasta and tomato sauce.

MOM'S LASAGNA

Okay, so the truth is that this dish is kind of a pain to make. But—and this is a big "but"—it's not hard . . . just labor-intensive. It's also so good that it's worth that extra labor, and let me tell you: once that baby arrives there will be no puttering in the kitchen doing things like gently laying pasta sheets over layers of cheese and vegetables.

So my advice is to make it now. And then eat it straight from the pan with a whole bunch of garlic bread, and love every second of your peaceful pre-baby pasta-eating.

Serves 6 to 8 (the leftovers keep really well in the freezer)

FOR THE LASAGNA

1 pound lasagna noodles

2 garlic cloves, minced

1 small yellow onion, diced

1 cup mushrooms (whatever type you like), finely chopped

Olive oil

2 bags (about 1 ½ pounds) baby spinach leaves, finely chopped

2 pounds whole-milk ricotta cheese

¼ pound Parmesan, grated

3 large eggs, beaten

Salt and pepper, to taste

½ pound mozzarella, shredded

FOR THE SAUCE

3 garlic cloves, minced

1 small yellow onion, finely diced

Olive oil

24-ounce can diced tomatoes

24-ounce can tomato puree

1 teaspoon sugar

⅓ cup water

Salt and pepper, to taste

Preheat your oven to 350°F.

Bring a large pot of water to boil for the lasagna noodles.

Now, make the sauce. In a medium-size, heavy-bottomed pan, sauté the garlic and onion in olive oil. When the onion is translucent, add the diced tomatoes, tomato puree, sugar, water, and some salt and pepper. Lower the heat and simmer for at least half an hour.

Next up: the filling for the lasagna. In a medium saucepan, sauté a couple more minced garlic cloves, diced onion, and mushrooms in olive oil until everything is tender.

In a large mixing bowl, combine the onion/mushroom mixture with the spinach, ricotta, Parmesan, and eggs, as well as a dash of salt and pepper.

Cook the lasagna noodles in the pot of boiling water until al dente (they'll cook a little more in the oven, so it's best to have them slightly undercooked at this point). If you're using no-cook noodles, skip this step.

Now it's time to construct your dish. Lay four cooked noodles in the bottom of a baking dish, placing them close together.

Layer on some of the spinach/cheese mixture, then a generous sprinkling of the shredded mozzarella, then tomato sauce, and repeat until you've used up everything except for ½ cup of mozzarella.

Finish it off with a layer of tomato sauce topped with the remaining mozzarella.

Cover the pan with foil and bake for 40 minutes. Remove the foil and bake an additional 10 minutes.

Let the cooked lasagna rest about 10 minutes, so that it settles. Cut into squares, and serve.

LAST-MINUTE BISCUITS

These are called "last-minute biscuits" because I never plan to make them, exactly; I make them either because I'm setting out dinner and it occurs to me that biscuits would be really good with whatever I see on the table, or because I'm pregnant and suddenly realize: need biscuits. Right now. Fortunately, with this recipe I can realize this, and then be eating them about fifteen minutes later.

Makes 8 to 12 biscuits

2 cups flour (plus more for sprinkling)

4 teaspoons baking powder

½ teaspoon salt

4 tablespoons shortening

¾ cup milk

Preheat your oven to 450°F.

Sift together dry ingredients in a large bowl.

Using a pastry cutter or two knives, cut in the shortening until you get a pebbly texture. Then stir in the milk.

Turn the dough out onto a floured surface and, with lightly floured hands, knead 20 to 30 times, until the dough holds together and is slightly elastic.

Pat down the dough until it's about 1 ¼ inch thick, and then use a small glass to cut out circles (you'll get 8 to 12, depending on the size of the glass you use).

Place your biscuits on a lightly greased cookie sheet and bake in the oven for 12 to 15 minutes, or until golden.

MAKE IT DESSERT!

Mash up some strawberries with granulated sugar, layer the strawberry mixture and some whipped cream on top of the biscuits, and presto: best strawberry shortcake ever.

WATERMELON, TOMATO, AND BASIL SALAD

This salad is one of my favorite dishes to make during the summer. It's so easy and refreshing, and has such unexpected flavors—the salty feta is incredible against the sweet watermelon.

There are lots of interesting ways to mix up the presentation, if you're serving it to guests: try substituting red and yellow cherry tomatoes, or plate each person's salad individually by arranging two long (about 3 x 1) rectangles of watermelon atop a few tomato rounds, and then sprinkling over the rest of the ingredients. You can also add Kalamata olives and sliced cucumbers if you want to make the salad even more robust and flavorful.

Serves 2

2 cups watermelon chunks

2 tomatoes (1 red, 1 yellow is pretty), sliced

⅓ cup crumbled feta cheese (make sure it's pasteurized)

Large handful of basil, roughly chopped

¼ cup olive oil

Sea Salt, to taste

Toss all the ingredients together in a large bowl and serve.

THE BEST SANDWICH IN THE WHOLE WIDE WORLD

My favorite thing about this sandwich is telling people what's in it. I start listing the ingredients, and their eyes get wide, and when I finish the list they—and I mean without fail*—say the two following sentences:*

"That's insane. I want one."

Serves 1

2 tablespoons peanut butter	½ banana
1 tablespoon Fluffernutter	3 slices cooked best-quality bacon
1 tablespoon Nutella	1 teaspoon honey

On a slice of bread, layer the above. Top it all with a second slice of bread.

MAKE IT BETTER (YES, IT'S POSSIBLE)

You can eat this sandwich as is, but I think this is a prime opportunity to get a little extra crazy with it.

If you have a press, put the sandwich in for a few seconds, until the insides get a touch runny. If you don't have a press, melt a little butter in a pan and put in the sandwich. Cover the pan and let the sandwich fry for a few seconds, then flip it, re-cover, and fry the other side until just golden.

Oh my god.

I am a thirsty, thirsty lady when I am With Baby. You probably are, too, which is good. It's your body's way of telling you to drink up, because while you don't need to drink *more* water than the average person when you're pregnant, you do have to be extra-sure that you're drinking *enough*. Which most people don't.

WATER THYSELF

If you find that you have trouble making sure you get your daily recommended amount of H_2O (about eight to ten 8-ounce glasses), try these tricks:

START SMART: You can get crazy dehydrated over the course of a night's sleep, so remember to start in on the water right when you wake up. Keep a glass of water next to your bed for middle-of-the-night sipping, and make it a habit to fill it up again and drink the whole thing right when you open your eyes in the morning, even if you don't feel especially thirsty.

BOTTLE IT UP: You're going to be carrying around a bottle in a few months anyway, so why not get used to it now? Find a reusable water bottle that you love, and make it your personal security blanket.

DRINK UP BEFORE YOU EAT UP: Make drinking a glass of water a pre-meal ritual: it's not only an easy way to remember to get extra hydration, it's also excellent for digestion (and will likely inspire you to eat a little cleaner during your meal, which can't be a bad thing).

CHOOSE CARBONATED: If you're not a huge fan of water, you can do what I do and get all weird and obsessive about your SodaStream machine. Carbonated water is just as hydrating as regular water, provided that you shoot for a type with no added sodium (sodium has electrolytes, which are good, but too much can be not-so-hot for your health).

FIRE UP THE FLAVOR: Adding some cucumber slices, strawberry slices, or citrus slices to a pitcher of water is a great way to make it taste *way* more appealing.

EGG CREAM

I grew up drinking egg creams, but apparently that's because I grew up in New York City. It appears that egg creams are something of a rarity in other parts of the world (or at least that's how it appears to me when I mention egg creams to people and am greeted more often than not with an expression that wouldn't be an inappropriate response to the statement, "I just ate a bunny rabbit"). Egg creams don't have eggs in them. They are not especially creamy. They are, however, awesome. They're basically ice cream sodas minus the ice cream, which may sound sad and disappointing, but is not. Promise.

Serves 1

½ cup cold whole milk

1 cup seltzer water

2 tablespoons chocolate syrup (Fox's U-Bet syrup is the classic pick)

Pour the milk into a tall soda glass. Top with the seltzer and stir vigorously, until it gets all fizzy and develops a nice head of foam.

Slowly pour the chocolate syrup down the inside sides of the glass. Give it another stir, and drink immediately with a straw.

FRESH MINT LEMONADE

Lemon and lemon-related things are kind of phenomenal picks for pregnant women. They're delicious, flavorful, aid in digestion . . . and can help to settle your stomach, which is especially nice right at the beginning and for those last couple of weeks before childbirth.

Now, the truth is that fresh-squeezed juices can be kind of a pain to make—I had to make fresh-squeezed orange juice every morning when I worked the brunch shift as a waitress in L.A., and it was misery from top to bottom—but once in a while? When you really, really want one? It's so *delicious, and totally worth a little extra trouble.*

Serves 2

¼ cup sugar

6 to 8 lemons

Small handful of mint leaves, chopped

In a small saucepan, combine the sugar and ¼ cup water. Bring it to a low boil and stir until the sugar has dissolved. Remove from the heat.

Squeeze the lemons (you should get about a cup of juice), reserving a few slices for garnish.

Fill a pitcher halfway with ice, and add the sugar water, lemon juice, chopped mint, and about two more cups of water. Mix and serve with lemon slices for garnish.

STRAWBERRY-BASIL FIZZ

And now: I would like to introduce you to your Pregnancy Mocktail.
This is what you get to make for yourself when you have guests over
and everyone's drinking their Blue Moons and their martinis and what
have you. Because you deserve something special, too, you get this.
(And just watch: everyone will totally want to try it and be kind of
jealous that they don't get their own Strawberry-Basil Fizz, too.)

Serves 1

3 or 4 large strawberries

Small handful of basil leaves

1 lime

1 cup club soda

Muddle the strawberries and basil leaves in a mortar and pestle (or in a
large glass using the back of a spoon).

Put the muddled strawberries and basil into a glass and fill it with ice.

Add a squeeze of fresh lime juice, then fill with club soda and stir
lightly.

Serve with an extra basil leaf and strawberry slice for garnish.

AMP IT UP (FOR THE OTHERS)

If you want to serve this to your other guests as a "real"
drink, just add one and a half ounces of Campari to each
serving and stir lightly.

When you get into your third trimester, the amount of advice that people have to offer you will all of a sudden dial up to the "unbearable" level. And one thing that every single one of them will inexplicably advise you to do is whip up a whole bunch of meals and divide them up into freezer bags so that all you have to do for dinner during those busy post-birth days is defrost a couple of portions in the microwave.

I say that's what Chinese food is for.

But one thing that I *do* think you should do is this: find the time to bake a handful of loaf cakes to stick in the freezer and defrost as needed. My rationale for this crazy-sounding piece of advice: loaf cakes are so delicious, and so useful. They make excellent breakfasts, snacks, and desserts, and even, when eaten in bulk, meal replacements (if you are capable of pretending, as I am, that cake = balanced meal, because there are eggs in there somewhere). And you will be so happy that you have freshly baked goods on hand when it is three in the morning and you've been bouncing your infant for two straight hours and there is nothing good on TV and your bangs are doing a weird vertical thing and you start thinking about how your hair will never ever again look like anything other than a tumbleweed because you will never ever again have a free hand with which to hold a hairbrush . . . and then abracadabra:

Cake.

Make the cake. You'll be happy you did. (So will the friends and family members who arrive to gaze upon your child and who forget that the golden rule of visiting a new parent is Bring Food.)

BASIC LOAF CAKE
Makes 1 loaf (8 to 10 slices)

1 ½ cups flour

2 teaspoons baking soda

¼ teaspoon salt

6 tablespoons butter

1 cup white sugar

2 large eggs

½ cup milk

Add-ins (see below)

Preheat your oven to 350°F.

In a medium-size bowl, combine the first three ingredients.

In a large bowl, cream together the butter and sugar. Add the eggs one at a time, mixing thoroughly between additions.

Gradually mix the dry ingredients into the butter/sugar mixture. Add the milk; mix well.

Mix in your add-ins (see box).

Pour the batter into a lightly greased loaf pan and bake for about 55 minutes, or until a toothpick inserted in the center comes out clean. Let cool before adding glaze or frosting, if using.

GET FANCY WITH IT

The fun thing about this cake is that you can make it taste like plain old cake (which is nothing to sneeze at) . . . or like anything else you might want, pretty much.

ORANGE-POPPY SEED CAKE: Before baking, add 1 tablespoon of finely grated orange zest and 2 tablespoons of poppy seeds. After baking, frost with chocolate icing and sprinkle a handful of chocolate chips over it for crunch.

LEMON CAKE: Before baking, add 1 ounce grated lemon zest. After baking, glaze with a mixture of 2 tablespoons lemon juice and $\frac{1}{4}$ cup of sugar.

RASPBERRY CAKE: Before baking, fold in 1 cup of frozen raspberries. After baking, top with a sprinkling of powdered sugar.

FREEZE!

1. Before freezing, cover the loaf in two layers of Saran Wrap and one layer of foil.

2. Store the loaf in the back of the freezer.

3. Defrost by setting it on a plate at room temperature or in the refrigerator.

4. Toast or warm individual slices in the microwave before serving (if there's any residual sogginess, toasting will get rid of it).

LET ME TELL YOU A LITTLE STORY about the very worst party in the world.

When I was twenty-five years old and living in Los Angeles, I discovered that my live-in boyfriend of a year and a half was cheating on me with a very pretty blonde actress. Unfortunately I also discovered that he was also cheating on that very pretty blonde actress . . . with me. Because he was her boyfriend, in addition to being mine.

This all came to a rather spectacular head on a beautiful June day when a friend of mine e-mailed me a photo of my boyfriend with his other-girlfriend. To say I was "upset" would be something of an understatement, but it actually turned into a rather enjoyable afternoon during which I reacted like I'd imagine any rational person would: I drank an entire bathtub's worth of Corona and blared Britney Spears while walking around the house collecting my boyfriend's possessions. Then I deposited them on my front porch, and called his mother and told her that she should probably come by to pick up her son's stuff before the trash collectors arrived in the morning to do the honors.

After the Corona/Britney Spears buzz wore off and the reality of what had happened sunk in, life got slightly less fun.

I wish I could say that in the following weeks I handled my heartbreak by being wonderfully resilient and deciding that I would no longer do things like invite terrible people into my life and then let them run amok through my emotions and home, but no. Instead, I dove headfirst into a period characterized primarily by a series of extremely poor decisions.

The party was one of them.

Shortly before the breakup I had made a new friend; let's call her "Tiffany." I met Tiffany at a club, and I liked her immediately. She was a Deep South girl with a huge head of wild blonde hair who screamed words rather than spoke them, and spending time with her was sort of like hanging out inside a bag of Pop Rocks. We got along famously, mostly because we were sort-of-to-very drunk about 100 percent of the time that we were together.

"LET'S DO THIS SHOT!"

"Okay!"

"LET'S DANCE ON THAT TABLE!"

"Yes!"

"LET'S PUT ON THAT MAN'S HAT AND THEN STEAL THE KEYS TO HIS HOTEL ROOM AND USE HIS HOT TUB AND EAT FRENCH FRIES IN IT."

"Tiffany, you have the BEST IDEAS EVERRR I LOVE YOUUU."

Summer heated up and Tiffany's birthday rolled around, so I offered to throw my new BFF a pool party at my place. "Invite some people over!" I said. "It'll be fun!"

The day of the party arrived, and all morning long things went smoothly. Five or six girls whom Tiffany had invited showed up, I put out guacamole in pretty bowls, and we all settled down around the pool with my little white dog snoozing nearby. At one point Tiffany emerged from my bedroom wearing a pirate costume complete with eye patch, thigh-high boots, and sword, but in the peaceful stillness of a perfect California morning that seemed more like a killer choice of attire than any indicator of the storm clouds brewing on the horizon. I climbed onto a raft and floated around, enjoying the sunshine and the sound of Gnarls Barkley coming from the stereo. It was lovely, and I felt like a very excellent friend and even more excellent pool party-thrower.

And then the doorbell rang. It was a few more of Tiffany's friends—two guys and a girl. Interestingly, they were also wearing pirate costumes. I started to sense that I had missed a key element of the party-planning process, but also couldn't see anything especially wrong with adding a theme to the afternoon, so I welcomed the newcomers in, and went back to my float and my sunshine.

Doorbell. More friends. More pirate costumes.

And then some more.

As it turned out, Tiffany had decided to advertise our little get-together* on MySpace. Now, you may not know a ton about MySpace if you are under the age of thirty, but let me tell you: it was quite the thing back in 2005. Everybody was on it, and so everybody—and I mean *everybody in the world*—showed up at my house. I knew exactly one of them, and she was pounding Hornitos tequila straight out of the bottle and swinging a sword

---

*Which had apparently been given the moniker "The Great Pirate Party."

around her head. I had invited only a couple of guests of my own, and neither of them had shown up yet.

When one of my invitees, a singer named Francesca who was a newish friend of mine, did eventually show up, what she walked into was not the chilled-out tropical luau that I had advertised, but rather a full-on rager complete with death metal blasting on the stereo, topless girls jumping into my pool, one boy whose idea of fun was to spend the better part of an hour body-slamming my glass-topped coffee table, and yet another who had diligently set himself to the task of writing on my furniture.

Writing. On my *furniture*.

Francesca stepped into my living room, took one look around, and walked straight out the side door, where she discovered me sitting on the stoop, rather calmly smoking a cigarette and petting my dog while I tried to figure out how in the world I was going to eject two hundred drunk lunatics from my home without calling the police, which for some reason felt at the time like an absolute last resort (*see*: period of life characterized by poor decision-making skills).

Now, Francesca is a very, very pretty, very girly-looking girl, with a china-doll face and brunette ringlets. On that particular day she was also wearing a white dress with a poofy skirt and little gold sandals, and so when she decided to take charge of the situation by marching into the very center of my living room, flicking off the music, and announcing to the guest of honor that her friends were to remove themselves from the premises *right now, please*, the effect that it had on Tiffany was essentially what you'd expect to see if Maria von Trapp declared to the monster living in Sigourney Weaver's refrigerator in *Ghostbusters* that he really should calm down, all that snorting and demonic roaring is terribly rude.

"There is no Tiffany. Only Zuul." Like that.

What Tiffany did next: lunged at Francesca, screamed into her face "YOU HAVE A BLACK SOUL AND DEAD EYES" (that's a direct quote), and pulled back a fist to hit her.

And so we grabbed my dog and ran.

How the whole thing came to an end: with myself and Francesca climbing out my bedroom window and hiding from Tiffany in the backyard while my friend Daniel—my second personal invitee, who had finally decided to make an appearance—somehow managed to funnel the Destructor and her merry band of furniture-tagging friends out my front door.

The Party from Hell ended up cementing a lifelong friendship between myself and Francesca, but other than that it was really not an especially ideal situation, what with the Magic Marker-ed tables, stolen money (oh, I didn't mention that part yet? Someone stole my wallet) and the hiding in an actual bush so that my guests wouldn't be able to find me.

Which is all to say: if your party goes south—as parties do, from time to time—don't do that.

Do this!

Entertaining for Adults

. . . .

WHEN YOU HAVE A BABY, you will no longer be interested in having parties that extend past 9:00 p.m. Maybe 8:00. Honestly, I'm pretty psyched when my parties close up shop around 6:00 or so, because that means I can both drink wine during the day and fall asleep at sundown.

Simple fact: late parties are just not on the agenda these days. The reason for this is that when you put a baby to sleep, he or she will be awake about two hours later, and then again two hours after that, and then again two hours after that. Even when the baby is no longer a baby, and becomes a full-on toddler, he or she will not understand the concept of sleeping past the rise of the sun, and you will find yourself desperately lurching toward your bed at the earliest possible second so that you can get something approximating a decent night's rest. Maybe. Not if you have dogs (*see*: page 170).

Which isn't to scare you. The other stuff that comes with parenthood is fun in a way that makes up for not sleeping. But it's important to go into this knowing beyond a shadow of a doubt that until your child becomes a teenager and never wants to get out of bed again, sleep will become such a precious-beyond-measure commodity that you will not sacrifice even one minute of it for a party that lasts beyond when it should.

When you're pregnant and exhausted from gestation-related matters (like a total inability to take a deep breath because your lungs have been pushed up into your neck somewhere) isn't a bad time to start practicing the party-ending technique that you will begin cultivating in earnest in just a few short months.

HOW-TO: END A GET-TOGETHER GRACEFULLY

Okay, so presumably the people you invited over aren't actually destroying your home or trying to punch you *à la* Tiffany. But everyone's been there: it's the end of the night, you're completely drained, and you still have a good couple of hours of cleaning ahead of you before you'll be able to collapse into bed . . . but a few guests just aren't quite ready to pack it up.

What to do?

Entertain early: The earlier you plan to start a party, the earlier you can plan to end it. I try to start my parties early enough that should a couple of my guests be interested in making it a late night, they can easily leave in time to make it somewhere else (a club, a bar, a party thrown by non-parent-type people) for the actual "nighttime" part of the evening. Later on that night, I will check out Instagram and "like" the photo of the fancy cocktail they drank at the cool bar they went to after leaving my place, and then I will fall asleep.

Announce the Start Time and the End Time: If you know that you'll want or need a party to wrap up by a certain time, make sure that the invitation (even if it's as informal as an e-mail) includes both a start and an end time ("Was thinking about having some people over this Saturday from 4:00 to 8:00 p.m. for cocktails and a light dinner—you interested?"). Your guests will likely be grateful for the heads-up, as it'll help them make their own arrangements for the rest of the day.

Clean it up: Clearing dishes and generally bustling around and straightening up (by which I mean wiping down the table as opposed to, say, breaking out the vacuum cleaner, which is a little too *get out of my house right now* for my taste) should be enough to inspire your guests to start collecting their things and heading on their way.

Be blunt: If you still have a couple of friends hanging around who just don't seem interested in taking off anytime soon and you're barely stifling those yawns, it's totally fine to be direct. A simple "I'm exhausted, I think I need to start wrapping things up" should do the trick without hurting any feelings.

Hand out goody bags: What, you thought these were for kids only? Nope. There is no one who does not enjoy being given a little present to take on their way, and the passing out of small "thanks for coming" gifts is a universally acknowledged symbol that the party has officially come to an end.

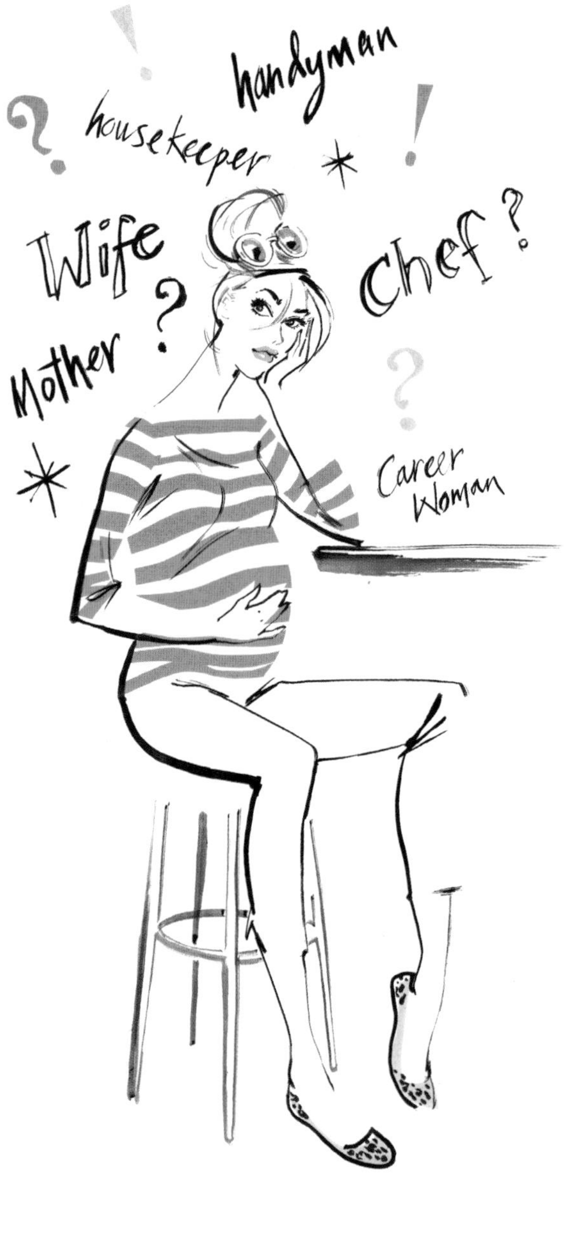

6

Relationships & Roller Coasters

(SHITTY DAYS, SECOND TAKES, AND WHAT TORI SPELLING TAUGHT ME)

I Hope You Have a Shitty Day

HORMONES ARE FUNNY THINGS. Except sometimes they're a little less funny, like when they almost get you arrested. Here's the thing: from time to time, I display a slight entitlement complex. That's okay; many of us do, especially now that social media functions to support our sincere belief that we are quite clearly the Most Important Person in the World ("My picture got liked eighty-seven times! I am *amazing*!"). Except my particular entitlement complex also leads me to believe that I am capable of talking my way out of virtually anything and everything. Because come on, what are they going to do . . . actually *say no*?

I don't think so.

Like this one time, when I was working at the law firm and managed to get the health insurance benefits for the entire company (all thirty or so employees, many of whom had families and various major medical issues for which health insurance is marginally important) sort of . . . canceled?

Guess what?

Got it back. Like a baller. (Mostly because the aforementioned certainty that I can talk my way out of anything and everything makes me *really* annoying to deal with if you are on the other side of all that talking, and I think the insurance company guy who ended up telling me that fine, we could have our insurance policy back honestly just wanted to get me off of the phone.)

Anyway, an unwillingness to stop talking until you are given your way is good sometimes, like when you've accidentally gotten a whole bunch of people's health insurance canceled. When you've lost your receipt and want to return something to a store with a no-returns-without-receipts policy. When you accidentally make an hour-long cell phone call from Canada without realizing that your contract doesn't cover that particular geographical locale, and would like the AT&T customer service rep to knock off that tiny little $300 charge, because come on, you didn't *mean* to do it.

. . . . Please?

It's maybe less good at other times, like when you park your car in the middle of a crosswalk on Madison Avenue because parking lots cost forty dollars *per hour* in that part of town and your husband has decided to take his sweet time exchanging a pair of sneakers while you sit wedged into the slightly-too-small-for-your-pregnant-self passenger's seat with your toddler in the back, thinking to yourself "If I am physically located inside the vehicle and my hazards are on, the decision to park in the crosswalk is, if perhaps not 'legal,' exactly, certainly the kind of only *semi*-illegal act that I will be able to talk my way out of." And then oops: here come the cops, and before you can catapult yourself into the driver's seat and speed away they've passed their blinky-thing over your registration sticker and handed you a ticket for $115.

That's what happened to me the other day. And that's also when the entitlement complex—which apparently gets slightly amped up in the presence of pregnancy hormones—kicked in.

So instead of doing what a person should probably do in that situation, which is apologize to the police officers for doing something that is, in retrospect, pretty unquestionably illegal, accepting my fine, and moving on with some degree of self-respect intact, I tried to sway them into a retraction by launching into an extremely detailed monologue during which I illuminated the fact that oh no, they didn't understand, what I was doing wasn't *parking* . . . it was *pausing.* And I can totally un-pause, right now! No problem!

And when that didn't work—like, at all? I got mad. The kind of mad that one should really never get at police officers, because they can do things like arrest you.

"THANKS VERY MUCH, officers. What NICE PEOPLE you are. I hope this makes you feel just FANTASTIC, giving a parking ticket to A PREGNANT WOMAN WITH A TODDLER."

Next step, when this resulted in being ignored rather than apologized to: a total abandonment of factual accuracy, aka "lying."

"I was just stopping for a minute!" Lie.

"To give my son a pretzel." Lie.

"And because I thought I felt a contraction." Oh, such a lying liar I am.

None of these worked, by the way, so I moved on to my *pièce de résistance*, and informed the officers that I would *not* be paying the ticket, I would *not* be returning to New York City (ever again!), and that on top of it all I sincerely hoped that they would have a shitty day.

I capped off my speech by ripping up the ticket into tiny pieces, throwing it down on the front seat of my car, and then announcing to Kendrick, who had just walked out of the sneaker store only to discover his pregnant wife strutting around like an angry peacock in front of two increasingly pissed-off police officers, "These people just *gave me a ticket*." As if the obvious thing that he needed to do was to defend my honor through any means necessary, up to and not necessarily excluding initiating a physical altercation. With police officers.

I pointed at the officers. "Say hi to the people who just *gave me a ticket*," I instructed Kendrick.

He said hi. And then he told me to get in the car and shut up. Which I did not do—or rather I did the first part, but certainly not the second—but to the policemens' credit, they moved along on their ticket-giving way, probably figuring that if my husband was making it through life with me, he probably didn't need any additional lecturing from the likes of them.

HOW-TO: TAKE A CHILL PILL

Being pregnant is stressful. The emotional roller coaster is real, and the last thing in the world that you want to hear is "It's just hormones." Which sure, it partially is, but there's also the little matter of all those massive physical changes that are taking place in your poor little body, so go ahead and let anyone who tells you "It's just hormones" know that nope, it's actually the fact that there is a child's foot lodged in your bladder. Ask them if that might stress *them* out a little. I bet you get a hug, if nothing else.

A few tried-and-true ways to chill out:

Morning hot water with lemon: If you're foregoing caffeine for the time being, you may miss those relaxing ten minutes you used to enjoy in the company of your coffee cup before your day began. Hot water with lemon makes for a wonderful (if slightly less exciting) morning ritual replacement. It's not only delicious and surprisingly eye-opening, but also aids in digestion (and yours may be a little sluggish these days thanks to—there they are again!—the hormones).

Lunchtime nap: If you can, make it a priority to catch a quick cat-nap during your lunch break. Even fifteen minutes can make a world of difference. If you have trouble shutting off, try one of those white noise apps on your computer or tablet. (RainyMood.com should honestly win an award of some sort.)

Evening stretch session: Taking just a few minutes every night to do some light stretching is not only crazy good for you (and can help with everything from pregnancy aches and pains to actual labor), it's awesomely relaxing—just make sure not to strain yourself; the point is to relax, not to get your Olympic gymnast on.

Mini-indulgences: Every day, try to treat yourself to something small: a mini-cannoli, a pretty new nail polish, or even just a few minutes alone doing absolutely nothing can be enough to make you feel like *you got this*. (Which you totally do.)

Exercise: Yeah, yeah. I don't like it, either. But during my first pregnancy I took just twenty minutes every day to bop around on an elliptical machine, and even though we're talking majorly low-im-pact (I barely even broke a sweat), it made a huge difference to how

I felt both physically and emotionally. It's just a fact: exercise makes you happier.

List-making: You know how they say that if you're having trouble falling asleep, you should write down everything on your mind on a notepad next to your bed to clear out the attic, as it were? Well, pregnancy is basically like that, except the things you're worrying about aren't "Pick up milk" but rather "Bring human life into world." There's a lot to worry about. Write it down; it helps.

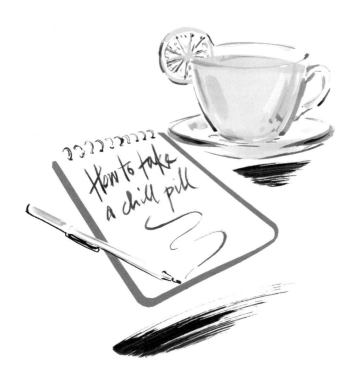

Way Back in the
Way-Back Beginning

. . . .

I WAS LYING IN BED, seven months pregnant, when Tori Spelling made me cry. I was watching an episode of *True Tori*: a reality miniseries in which Tori Spelling and her husband, Dean McDermott, deal with the aftermath of his infidelity. And while the subject matter obviously isn't the most uplifting topic in the world, I was still surprised to find myself actually in tears.

The episode in question revolved around a therapy session during which the couple explored Dean's "rationale" for cheating, and what the conversation quickly revealed was that he just didn't feel like he was getting enough sex in his marriage. The subtext: even if that didn't make his actions "right," didn't it make them a little more . . . understandable? . . . Maybe?

What *was* understandable: Tori's response to this, which was to break down in tears. She said that she had always known that he would cheat on her, because he was so focused on what their marriage had been like "in the beginning"—the implication being that they started out doing what many new couples do, which was have sex every day, or even multiple times a day—and that he would never be happy unless she kept that standard going. Forever.

"We had a great relationship and we had a great sex life," she said to her husband.

"We had sex once every two weeks," Dean shot back. "It wasn't fantastic."

And in response to this, their therapist expressed the sentiment that I suspect was on the mind of every single woman watching the show: "Dean," she said, "your expectation of what a marriage is supposed to be like sexually . . . it's like a fairy tale."

Let's get real: sex every other week is hardly cause to declare a State of Emergency for couples who have been together for many years, and who are raising young children (many might argue, in fact, that every other week ain't half bad). But the set of expectations that Tori's husband was working from makes perfect sense in a society where Real Housewives write books about how sex every other day (at a minimum!) is the only way to keep a marriage healthy, where celebrities appear in bikinis looking picture-perfect mere weeks after giving birth, where the message from every advertisement and every TV show and every magazine is that not only "can" you be a mom and a sex bomb, you *must* be, because if you are not you are just another woman who Got Married and Got Boring.

The message here, of course, is that if you fail to keep things "hot," any subsequent failure is on you. Because men are men and men need sex and sure, we'll all *tell* the woman who's busy working and raising children and exploring her personal interests and not being intimate with her husband as often as he (or she) might have liked because sometimes life gets in the way that it wasn't her fault that he sought out sex elsewhere, but inside we're thinking: "Well, it kind of . . . was. Wasn't it?"

I think mothers can—should—feel sexy. I think intimacy can—should—continue to be a wonderful, special, important part of a relationship during a pregnancy, and after the kids arrive.

But it's not always that simple, and not always that easy. The scene between Tori Spelling and her husband broke my heart because I understood exactly where she was coming from, the exact fear that she was dealing with and could not get away from and that haunted her every day.

I am different than I used to be, in so many ways, up to and including the degree to which I prioritize intimacy. And so I wonder: does being "different than I used to be" mean that I'm failing to uphold my end of the "deal"? Because that's how it feels, so much of the time. Like there was a deal that we made, and I broke it.

It's not even about sex; sex is such a small part of it. It's about all those things that were one way in the beginning, and are another way now. It's also not my husband who makes me feel this way; it's me. It's me who worries that I promised my partner one version of myself, and that now, many years and many life changes down the line, I'm simply not the same girl he signed on for. I look older. I feel older. I'm exhausted nearly all of the time. I wear sweatpants—and not the cute ones; the kinds that all sorts of Internet articles and relationship "experts" tell you never, ever to wear around your husband—around my husband. Because sweatpants are comfortable, and because adorable negligees are not, and because sometimes I just want to eat my Chinese food and watch my dumb reality show like a big lump on the couch and not worry about it.

Except I do. Worry about it.

A few weeks after Kendrick and I met, he came out to visit me in Los Angeles. We drove to Las Vegas and got engaged at three o'clock in the morning in a hotel room with gold-painted walls and a mirrored ceiling. On the way back to L.A., we stopped at a Ralph's supermarket and picked up a *Brides* magazine and hamburger meat and buns and blue cheese and cheap champagne, and we went back to my house and sat in my backyard and grilled burgers and couldn't keep our hands off of each other, and at one point he turned to me and said, "Can life always be just like this?"

And I said that yes, it could, and I meant it.

But at that moment, twenty-six years old and newly engaged to a man I barely knew, sitting by a pool in the California sunshine, I didn't know what I was promising.

At seven months' pregnant, all that I want to do is fall asleep the moment that I finally collapse into my bed at night. I want to sleep as long as I can, and as much as I can, and when I'm not sleeping or taking care of our two-year-old son I'm working or preparing a nursery for our unborn daughter or cooking or vacuuming up whatever horrible thing our dogs just left in our living room . . . and where, exactly, does intimacy figure into all of that?

Sometimes it feels like I don't even know.

And it's not only since I've been pregnant. The moment that I became a mother, something changed. It's not that I feel "unsexy"; it's not that I don't "like" my postpartum (or pregnant) body or that I worry that my husband doesn't like it; it's not that I feel guilty about sexuality or afraid or distant or any of the other things that my pregnancy books warn me about . . . it's that the part of me that feels like a responsible grown-up who's got to Get Stuff Done and the part of me that feels like a fun-loving, carefree girl who's up for anything, anywhere, wherever and whenever sometimes seem completely at odds with each other, like there's no room for both women in my one little body.

I went into motherhood absolutely committed to the idea that I'd keep my "wife" self and my "mom" self separate. I had this fantasy that once our children were in bed and our responsibilities for the day had ended we'd return to who we'd always been: that couple who couldn't keep their hands off of each other, who chased each other around the house and acted like kids and viewed intimacy not as another mark on the to-do list, but as an addiction.

In my mid-twenties, during a period when I was busy trying to figure out what I wanted to do with my life and not doing a very good job of it, I spent a few months working at the Meatpacking District bar that the movie *Coyote Ugly* was based on. My "work uniform" was a bikini top and cutoffs. My job requirements included dancing on top of the bar, pouring whiskey down customers' throats, and singing Creedence Clearwater Revival into a megaphone. The lines between what I did to make money and what I did to have fun were so blurry they were nearly invisible: as my shift came to an end, my friends streamed in to order beers and drop quarters into the jukebox, and my husband spent the afternoons when he didn't have band practice camped out at the end of the bar, watching me slam the heels of my cowboy boots into the wood in time to the music. My work was all about freedom and debauchery, letting loose and letting go, and so in those days my sexuality seemed to come along with me wherever I went. It wasn't a part of me that I had to "unleash" at some appropriate hour after the workday had come to an end and I could unbutton my suit jacket and strip off my tights; it just *was*.

Now my days are spent running from meetings to music classes to playgrounds, and by the time the day rolls to a close and I've read one more bedtime story and changed one more diaper and brought one more glass of water into a room filled with Thomas the Tank Engines and stuffed animals, I'm not quite sure how to turn around and dance back into my old self.

My husband and I used to spend all day in bed together in a big tangle of sheets, nothing to do but pick up a phone and order another pizza. And now I want to get into that bed and sleep, and sleep, and if I've gotten enough sleep, which I never do, I want to read a book, or surf around on the Internet. I want to wake up with the sun, jump off of stone walls yelling "Superman!" with my son, and one day help my daughter figure out the difference between a triangle and a square. I want to *want* to light candles and eat pasta in bed on a Sunday afternoon and find that time that is just for my husband and me . . . but right now, I don't know where I'd even start looking for it, because there is *so much else to do.* And that scares me.

Because I can't help but remember that day when my husband asked me if life could always be this way, and feel like I lied. Sure, he was asking about hamburgers and champagne and making even the smallest moments feel like celebrations, but really: wasn't what he was asking about *us*? Would *we* always be that way?

We would not. We would change, and then change some more, and eventually change so much that it would be hard to even remember that we used to be those kids sitting in the backyard with ketchup in their hair.

And so when I saw that episode of *True Tori*, I cried. Because it was one of my greatest fears come to life: that the changes that come to be in any marriage, those up-and-downs that are an inevitable part of weeks and months and years spent in the company of another person, wouldn't be okay with my partner. They'd make him feel cheated, like he'd been promised one thing and given another, and they'd eventually bring our partnership—and, worst of all, our *family*—to an end.

Here's where it gets even more complicated: sometimes, I feel like the ways in which I've changed mean I've broken a promise I made not only to my partner, but to myself, and all the worry and the guilt makes it hard to see what I even really enjoy. Most days, I want to put on makeup that makes me feel pretty, or wear a pair of heels that make me feel glamorous. I feel strongly that those things have a place in my life that is good and exciting and based in empowerment rather than a sense of inadequacy. But on other days I *don't* want to put on makeup, or wear heels . . . and sometimes I feel that I have to anyway, because if I don't, I worry about what it might mean about promises made and then broken.

And so I wonder: how can I believe that it is important to do those things that make me feel like I might still be a girl even though I mostly feel like a mother, and yet feel burdened by the sense that I *have* to do it all, be it all. All things to all people, all at once, all of the time?

Isn't that enormously, almost cripplingly inconsistent? It is. And that inconsistency makes sense.

Because there are enormous, almost crippling inconsistencies in how society positions women and mothers. It's not just that society expects us to "do it all," it's that the things that it wants and expects us to do often act in total opposition to each other.

Society pressures women to be sexy, and expects women to

be note-perfect mothers, but does not want them to be sexual creatures and mothers at the same time. It tells us that we must put our children above everything, but also that while it's maybe not technically our fault if we don't have sex with our husbands every day and they cheat on us . . . it kinda is.

The expectations placed upon us aren't just "high"—they are fundamentally opposed *to themselves*, and are thus not just "tough," but actually impossible to uphold. And if you are struggling—as I am—with figuring out how to be all of the things that you want to be, all at the same time, that simple fact—if nothing else—should make you feel so much better.

It's impossible.

And that's okay. You are okay. Even if you don't feel like being "sexy" today; even if you do. Because when you partner up with someone for the whole of Forever, evolution isn't only inevitable, it's necessary. Exciting. And becoming a parent is the greatest evolution of all, and it is going to result in changes: changes you're happy about; changes you're not; changes that just are, because there's no other way to be.

That feeling that you had in Week One with your partner— that crazy, wild, can't-get-enough feeling—that's so much fun, of course it is, and there are threads of that intoxication that will trail through your relationship forever, but that's also such a narrow scratch on the surface of what you get when what you get is a lifetime. The beauty isn't in the champagne; it's in the moments when you're cleaning up the dishes after your guests have left, standing next to each other in the kitchen scrubbing at some pots, and you realize that this is the most fun you've had all night: just the two of you all alone in an empty room after the party is over, laughing at the same unsaid joke.

So here is what I am asking you to do: talk to your partner about what's going on in your mind, whatever it may be. Delete the Internet articles that say that you shouldn't wear sweatpants around the house, go put on your biggest, ugliest pair, and then sit down on the sofa and *tell your partner what scares you*. Parenthood changes everyone involved—not just the person who physically gave birth—and I'm willing to bet that your worries will be met with understanding, appreciation, compassion, and a few worries of your partner's own.

And even if they're not? Even if you lay bare your greatest fears and your admissions are met with frustration, confusion, and inflexibility?

Guess what? More change is still to come. It's a long road that we have ahead of us as lovers, as partners, and as parents, and the only thing that's certain is that nearly everything will turn out in a way other than what we imagined.

What's important isn't to stick around in the way-back beginning; how it was when you first met was nice and all, I'm sure, but it was also the past.

And the future is what's worth fighting for.

Ur Doing It Wrong

· · · · · · · · · · ·

WHEN YOU ARE PREGNANT, you get a lot of unsolicited advice. When you are pregnant and talk about being pregnant on the Internet, you get what amounts to a tidal wave of UR DOING IT WRONG.

Among the things I have "done wrong" as a parent, according to people I both do and do not know:

- Had a baby, generally
- Had a baby and did not immediately have another baby
- Had another baby
- Breast-fed in public
- Didn't breast-feed for long enough, in public or otherwise
- Worked from home
- Worked outside of the home
- Put socks on my baby
- Forgot to put socks on my baby
- Exercised
- Not exercised
- Put a hat on my baby, but not sunglasses (because a hat is not enough)
- Put sunglasses on my baby (because they can poke him in the eye)
- Owned a rug (because he can slip)
- Did not own a rug (because he can fall)

- Permitted my toddler to have a lollipop
- Permitted my toddler to have another applesauce
- Bought my toddler this kind of juice, not that kind
- Bought my toddler that kind of food, not this kind
- Did my own thing and tried not to worry about people judging me for how I was raising my baby
- Worried about people judging me for how I was raising my baby

You cannot win. And you should not try, because everyone who's ever been pregnant or who's known someone who's been pregnant has an opinion about the optimal way to gestate, and if you listen to everyone's shoulds and should-nots you'll A) go crazy, and B) end up not listening to *yourself*, which is the person you should be listening to (in addition to your doctor, of course).

As an example, let's go back to the topic of exercise. This is a subject on which I should probably not opine, 'cause my version of exercise is, like I said, more akin to "making soft and gentle leg motions while devoting 90 percent of my energy to reading *US Weekly* and checking my text messages," but bear with me.

When you say the word "exercise" and you are expecting, people get very, very serious about what you absolutely must and must not do. I have been spotted walking down the street and been told that I need to move more slowly so as not to over-exert myself (it's bad for the baby). I have also been instructed to exercise every day, but not in that way (also bad for the baby) or in this way (so, so bad for the baby), but rather only in this very specific way that is good for the baby. Which is a way that someone else told me is bad for the baby.

This is all people just trying to be helpful, of course, but the end result of all this noise is the danger that I will lose my ability to listen to what the body that's gotten me this far is telling me. Which, in this case, is that—as much as I hate to admit it—some kinds of exercise actually feel pretty good. And other kinds of exercise feel bad, and it's all very particular to me and my lifestyle—just like it'll be particular to you and your lifestyle, and that's just fine.

Something else that's just fine: wondering whether everything is just fine. There will be those who tell you "not to let any negative thoughts seep in" when you're pregnant, as if worry is a cheeseburger that will pass directly through the umbilical cord and into the mouth of your hungry little fetus. Again, well-intentioned, but this kind of attitude makes women feel scared to express their feelings, lest others judge them for not having the "right" kinds of emotions, and fear like this is not only hurtful—it's dangerous. Because it makes you feel like you can't say "I'm scared" or "I'm anxious" or "I need help" . . . and being able to say that you need help is the first step toward actually getting it.

In italics, because this one is important: *it is okay to feel nervous, scared, anxious, or insecure when pregnant*. This is an enormous adjustment both physically and emotionally, and it's only natural that with all the positive feelings come some ambivalent (or even negative) ones. If you resent your body's newfound aches and pains, if you're having trouble feeling a connection to the baby while he's still in your tummy, if you just really want the whole pregnancy period to be over and done with so you can get to the mothering part already . . . all these things are okay, and don't mean that you'll be a terrible parent. Don't let anyone make you feel bad for having less-than-sunny moments, and if you're feeling *really* bad, talk to someone, whether that's a friend, a family member, or a professional.

And when someone instructs you to buck up, that feeling down is bad for the baby, go ahead and tell them that Jordan says that when she was pregnant with her daughter she once got so upset with her husband because he had an expression on his face that she interpreted as "I do not love you" when what it actually meant was "there is mold in the jelly and that makes me mad because I want to eat jelly" that she flailed around in hysterics to the point where she jammed her finger on the staircase and ended up sitting on the toilet seat crying while bandaging her sad, jammed hand, and her baby is just fine.

Someone with Problems

Growing up, my parents taught me that no one would handle my problems for me; it was on me to face them, and then fix them. If I had an issue with a teacher, a fight with a friend, an essay that I just couldn't seem to get right, they were there to listen and offer suggestions, of course, but they were not going to storm the gates and take over; finding a solution was my job. And I'm grateful for that.

A strange by-product of this focus on self-reliance, though, is the fact that my family—myself included, as it turns out—doesn't really believe in medication. Tylenol for a headache, Lipitor for cholesterol, sure . . . but drugs for the mind? Nope. Maybe it's a generational thing; maybe it's pride; maybe it's a reaction to the rampant overmedication going on in today's society, but whatever it is, my family's attitude toward psychiatric medications (and therapy in general) burrowed itself deeply into my head. So deeply that despite the fact that I like to think that I'm a generally open-minded person—and think that if something hurts, you should look for ways to fix it—I grew up believing that (barring "serious" mental disorders like schizophrenia, bipolar disorder, aka "things that happen to other people"), you do not need pills to fix your head.

You should be stronger than that.

Or at least *I* should be.

The strangest part: I studied cognitive neuroscience (basically, the biology underlying psychological behavior) in college, which means that I know better than this, am more educated about the very real neural mechanisms that contribute to psychological conditions than the average bear. In particular, I spent a lot of my college career studying so-called "shadow syndromes"—the milder forms of major mental disorders that plague so many of us and go untreated because they aren't as showy as their more dramatic cousins—and I know that these syndromes are real, and cause real problems in people's lives. I know that highly effective medications have been developed to address them.

And still: part of me thought that for a "normal" person (such as myself, I suppose, although I also know better than to toss around the word "normal") to take a pill for depression or anxiety (both issues that virtually everyone deals with)—was . . . lazy. "The easy way out."

"I'm smart," I thought. "I'm self-aware. I can handle a little anxiety."

I was wrong, both about the fact that my anxiety was "little" and about the fact that I could tackle it with my own bare hands, but it took me a good ten years to figure this out. And what finally did the trick was admitting to myself once and for all that what I was experiencing was way, way off the spectrum of what can be considered "normal" (because, of course, some degree of anxiety is not only unavoidable; it's actually beneficial, helping us run away from bears we encounter in the woods and such). My anxiety, I finally came to understand, was pathological: it disrupted my sleep, my relationships, my *life*. It wasn't something that I should or could just "deal with."

I guess I finally just got sick of feeling this way.

A couple of weeks postpartum, I was prescribed a low-dose medication to combat the chronic insomnia and anxiety that I'd been dealing with for a good decade (and hopefully make PPD more unlikely), and the turnaround that I experienced was extreme enough that I now feel comfortable saying that my decision to finally try medication is one of the best decisions that I have ever made in my life. That's not an exaggeration.

What was I so afraid of? I suppose I was afraid that I would feel "drugged," that the medication would dull my feelings and my emotions and leave me something other than myself. I was terrified that my children would grow up with a shell of a mother, looking out at the world with glassy eyes that never quite saw them. Dramatic, maybe, but that's what I pictured. But what I experienced was no dulling of the emotions at all. I'd describe it, rather, as a sharpening of reality, with the noise of "what-if" replaced by the solid steadiness of what *is*.

I am still stressed. I am still worried. I still get frustrated. I still get angry. But I am not overwhelmed by these feelings. They feel, for the first time in as long as I can remember, ordinary. Like rational responses to the world around me. They feel manageable.

My worries used to scream so loudly inside my head that I couldn't hear anything else—certainly not anything approaching logic—but now, for the first time in as long as I can remember, I'm able to hold a fear in my mind, turn it over and examine it, and then either deal with it or put it away on a shelf, to be explored at some later date. Far from feeling drugged, I feel clearer than I have felt in years. And the effect that this clarity has had on my life—and especially my marriage—has been nothing short of remarkable. I can worry about work, and then put aside the worry and play with my son before he goes to bed. I can argue with Kendrick and explain my feelings rather than lashing out.

I can let it—whatever "it" is—go.

I was also afraid of something else, something even more frightening: that taking a pill would mean that I was altering my identity, somehow changing my label in this world from Someone Who's Got It Under Control to Someone With Problems. But then, after I wrote a post in which I talked about my decision to explore medication, I got so many e-mails from readers saying that they struggled with anxiety but were fearful of the stigma of talking about it, and especially feared having others discover that they were seeking medical help . . . and I realized that the fact that I'm scared of that stigma, too, is exactly why I need to be open about it.

You know, I'm not saying that the perspective that I had growing up was "bad," not at all. It taught me how to do the hard work that goes into confronting problems rather than skimming over the surface and seeking out miracles. And I think it's even what ultimately allowed me to make this change now, to overturn a belief so deeply rooted that it couldn't even be shifted by years of education in the cold, hard facts about psychological disorders.

I see now that I spent years determined to fight a battle with my bare hands instead of looking around me for other tools that I not only "could" use, but were, in fact, necessary. So maybe it's not an overhaul of my belief system at all, but rather an evolution: a focus not on self-reliance to the point of "I got this" hubris, but rather on finding a solution to the problem, whatever that may be.

There is a difference between a crutch and a tool; one shoulders the burden for you, perhaps keeping you from building up the strength to carry it yourself . . . and the other just makes you stronger.

The Second Time Around

. . . .

I WASN'T SURE I wanted to have a second child. And then all of a sudden I was. Not sure that we were "ready"—I'd never be sure of that—but sure that I wanted to move on to the next place we were headed. Sure that I wanted to meet the newest member of our family.

During my first pregnancy, I thought about it for what felt like every minute of every day. I read websites, researched products, made lists, knitted blankets, wrote e-mail after e-mail after e-mail to my mother about stroller options and car seat options and coming-home-from-the-hospital outfit options. I did stretches every single night before bed for half an hour, remembered to take my prenatal vitamin every morning, carefully cataloged my doctor's appointments, rubbed oils into my skin, spent time putting together cute maternity outfits and made five trips to Buy Buy Baby before finally deciding which color baby carrier was my favorite. Most nights, when I walked home from the subway station, I went several blocks out of my way to buy my favorite cupcake from my favorite cupcake shop.

Being pregnant, take two, is a different animal.

Like the other day, I wanted a cannoli. Third-trimester-style wanted it (which is a lot of wanting it). And I was going to hop in the car and get one, but first my son wanted some macaroni and cheese, so I made that. And then I remembered that I had to call the pediatrician, and cancel a play date, and pick up a toy for my son's friend's birthday party, and while at the toy store I spent really a lot of time explaining to my son that he already has that fifteen-dollar plastic stegosaurus at home, so let's go ahead and unhand it minus the tears, please. And then it was 6:00 p.m. and too late to start dinner, so I ordered a pizza and put some frozen broccoli in the microwave so that I could pretend that what was about to happen was that we were going to eat a balanced meal. And then it was bath time, and story time, and bedtime, and then my bedtime because I could not stand up straight for one more second, and: oh right. The cannoli.

. . . Maybe tomorrow?

When I found out I was pregnant with my first baby, everyone told me that buying burp cloths with cute elephants on them didn't matter, that having the exact stroller of my dreams didn't matter, that whether or not my nursery looked straight out of a Pottery Barn catalog didn't matter . . . and I half-listened, and half-*yeah yeah yeah*-ed while I went right ahead and did what I wanted to do anyway, because no matter what they said, I still thought it mattered. And as much as I hate to admit this:

They were right.

The burp cloths, the stroller, the nursery, it's all fun and there's nothing wrong with caring about things for no reason larger than the fact that they make you happy, but it's also all for *you*. Which means that if these thing *aren't* making you happy—if all that planning and designing and organizing and arranging just-so—is making you crazy, you can skip it. If you don't feel like painting tiny stencils onto the borders of the nursery walls and would really rather sit down for a second in a dark room with a Sprite and take a break from all of it—the pregnancy, the lists, the baby on the way, the nursery that has yet to be finished? Do that instead. Stencils are cute. They also do not matter to the baby one tiny bit.

For some people, putting on a little makeup and a pair of heels is a mood-lifter, and for others it's nothing but a pain. I'm usually firmly planted in that first category, but for pregnancy number two I found myself in the second much of the time, because the vast majority of my head space was being taken up by things like making sure that my son didn't fall off of that play structure and calling Time Warner because no, we didn't order *Guardians of the Galaxy* sixteen times (only twelve) and trying to get finger paint (which they said was washable but apparently they lied) out of a Baby Gap jean jacket. And what this 180-degree attitude shift made me realize was maybe most reassuring of all.

It's so important to incorporate the small things that make you happy into your life in whatever ways you can, but it's also important to remember that *what makes you happy is allowed to change over time*. You can care about having a brand-new stroller with a space-age cup holder for one baby, and just borrow your sister's beat-up Baby Jogger for the next, and still love both your children just the same. You can care about cute maternity outfits today, and not give a snack pack about what you look like tomorrow.

You can evolve, and have a second pregnancy that looks in no way like the first, and what that means about your love for either child is exactly nothing.

The first time around, I spent all nine months relaxing and pampering myself and feeling kind of like a magical pregnancy unicorn. This time, what I feel like is more akin to "miserable, all of the time." With pregnancy number two, as it turns out, instead of reclining on a pillow and watching *The View*, you're finding space on your nonexistent lap for a toddler who wants you to read him a story. You're figuring out how to pick up thirty pounds of child with a nice dose of sciatica paralyzing your lower body. You're waking up at 6:00 a.m. instead of doing what you want to do, which is not get out of bed at all until someone comes to wake you up with pancakes. And you don't get cannolis. Ever. If you want something sweet, what you get are the sad, weird-shaped white-and-orange marshmallows that are left in your toddler's bowl of Lucky Charms after he's eaten up all the clovers and rainbows.

The first time around, I thought a lot about the "stuff" that came along with being pregnant. This time, I know where all that stuff is heading: half of it is going to end up at a yard sale, being sold at a depressing discount, and the other half is going to end up being vomited on so often that it turns frightening colors and has to be thrown out. And when it comes to choosing a stroller? Please. I'll take that one, because it is closer to me than the one over there and I am too tired to think about wheel-locking mechanisms for even one more second.

But with a second pregnancy, there's also this: you know what it feels like to fall in love, and you can't believe that very soon you'll get the chance to do it again. When you know what's on the horizon, and that what's on the horizon is a love that will outpace anything you've ever felt before in your life by leaps and miles, you realize that while a car seat in your favorite color can brighten your day, the fact that your budget only accommodates the less expensive model in the less-cute color won't matter one bit, because you also know that when all is said and done you won't be looking at the seat at all. You'll just be seeing the person inside it.

The Space Between

. . . .

THERE WAS A TIME, about five years ago, when my husband and I fought and fought, and it felt like the fighting would never stop. It was a time when it seemed like anything that could go wrong did (and would continue to forever and ever); Kendrick's band—the band he'd devoted the entirety of his post-college life to—was coming apart at the seams; I'd been fired by my acting agent and was spending my days working at a job that I hated; we had no money and a too-small apartment and drank too much cheap wine and talked too little, and when we tried to look into our future, we couldn't see where the disappointment—or the fighting—would ever end. When we fought, we didn't fight with the hope that we'd arrive at some kind of resolution. The goal was nothing more than to prove that the other was at fault.

Things are bad, we each said, *and you are why.*

I can't even remember the things we were "actually" fighting about back in those days. It could have been the dishes, or who last took the dogs for a walk; it didn't matter, because once we got going the fights spiraled off in any direction they could, quickly landing us both in a place where we couldn't even hear the words that the other was saying because our heads were so filled with rights and wrongs and blame.

It felt like I was going backward to the person I'd been years ago, when I lived in Los Angeles and hadn't liked myself very much, and like there was nothing we could do to stop ourselves from falling even further away from each other. I felt toxic, poisoned, like my very bones left me incapable of being the kind of person in a relationship who I dreamed of being: thoughtful, respectful. Kind. Willing to listen.

But things changed. I didn't think they could, or would . . . but they did.

Everybody fights. *Everybody.* Whenever you put two people with different backgrounds, values, and approaches to life in the same living space and then tell them to spend a concentrated amount of time together every single day, they are going to fight. So the question is not "whether" you fight; it's "how" you fight. Kendrick and I fought badly, but we wanted to learn how to fight better. And if we were going to have a family together, it wasn't just "a good thing to do." It was everything.

One night right in the middle of the summer, the fight got so big that it felt like it would take down everything from our marriage to the very walls around us. The fight that we had that night was about so many things—big things, small things, but mostly just the fact that we were so unhappy. We argued for hours—Kendrick pacing the living room, picking things up and putting them down again, me sitting cross-legged on the floor in an old T-shirt—and were finally so tired and overwhelmed that we just gave up and said what we meant, and what we meant was this:

I do not like how things are and I want them to be better and I don't know how to do that and I'm scared.

Once we both admitted that things needed to change and that neither of us had any idea how to change them—but that we did know that we wanted to change them together rather than apart—that's what made the difference. We wanted to pull ourselves back from the edge, and so we had to do our best to make our future together—not "winning," or proving the other person "wrong"—our priority.

God, are relationships ever a lot of work.

When I lived in Los Angeles I had an ex-boyfriend who said a lot of terrible things to me, but I think that the worst thing that he ever said, the thing that let me know once and for all that our relationship was doomed, was that he did not believe that relationships should be work. He said that they should be easy, and that the people in them should not have to "try." He was wrong.

You don't just have to "work" in a relationship . . . you have to *keep working*. All the time, and especially when your life gets turned upside down.

And when it does, remember this: fighting without reason and without end? It's so often a problem that lies in the space between: the space where the truth is getting lost in all those emotions and all those words.

What matters is not that you don't fight, but that you're both committed to seeing your way out the other side, to making it through the rough patches together, and to *listening to each other*. It's the most important thing you can do: just listen. Let your partner know they're being heard. And make sure that you have a voice as well.

Kids

. . . .

I LIKE TO SAY I was a "good kid" growing up, but it was more complicated than that. Like the girl in the rhyme, I was good when I wanted to be, and when I was bad I was, if not "horrid," exactly, certainly no angel.

On the one hand, I had all the Type A trappings (and neuroses) that you'd expect from a little girl who grew up attending fancy New York City private schools that encouraged her to pick an Ivy League to aspire to at the ripe old age of six. I got mostly As and A minuses; I read *Ulysses* cover to cover at sixteen; I was the head of the Curriculum Committee and never, ever showed up late for play rehearsals. I had a bank account with savings that I had made myself through my acting jobs, wrote papers the night they were assigned rather than the night before they were due, and (this is true) read every single word in every single book ever assigned to me throughout the entirety of my academic career, memorizing large passages of text prior to every test so that I would be able to effortlessly regurgitate on command not just the "correct" answer, but the "perfect" one. I was terrified of failure in a way that made me err way on the side of getting things done, and getting them done well.

Perfectly, I hoped.

But I also roamed Central Park after dark nervously drinking wine spritzers alongside teenagers who I wanted—so badly—to be my friends but were really just kids who I sort of knew. They had spiked-up, blue-and-purple-dyed hair, did drugs with names I'd never heard before, and gave themselves heart tattoos on their calves with homemade kits at two in the morning. We would sit in circles in the center of Sheep Meadow, only getting up to run away from the cops' searchlights, or stand in bunches outside the Burger King on the Upper West Side, or drape ourselves over couches at whoever's place was empty of parents for the evening. We smoked clove cigarettes in townhouse stairways, and crushed up Ritalin pills on Crate & Barrel dressers.

I felt nervous around my friends, but somehow less nervous around my boyfriends, so jumping from one bad romantic decision to another usually felt like the easiest thing to do. I dated a pothead who spent his afternoons (and weekends, and school days) rolling blunts and watching *The Doors*; a pale, skinny Billy Corgan wannabe who simultaneously dated my friend and liked grabbing my arm too hard; an aspiring mechanic who ran away from home to live in a rooming house in Maine with some heroin-addict buddies and, as I discovered when I checked up on him on Facebook nearly two decades later, ended up in exactly the same place where he'd started.

There was a movie called *Kids* made in the 1990s by a guy named Larry Clark, about a single night in the lives of a group of high schoolers with very little to do other than walk around New York City in search of problems that feel like fun. The movie wasn't only a fairly accurate depiction of the things that the teenagers I was hanging around with were up to; the casting director actually plucked several cast members straight from our ranks. Not me, of course—I was terrified of things like sex and drugs, and hardly gave off a "bad girl" vibe—but I made it my business to be *around* things that frightened me whenever I could. I couldn't believe how little thought the people I hung around with gave to what they put into their bodies and what came out of their mouths, and I suppose part of me hoped that a dose of all that not-caring might flow into me by virtue of proximity.

Caring a little less would have been nice.

One summer, most of my friends went off to country homes in Vermont or to camp. I didn't have a summer home, and I didn't like camp, so I stayed in the hot, empty city, taking the M11 bus up Amsterdam Avenue and then back down Columbus, stopping off at Barnes & Noble to sit cross-legged on the floor and read books about witchcraft for a while before going home to light some candles and stare into the pendulum that my aunt had given me, hoping that it would tell me something.

In August my friends came back, and we resumed our busy schedule of standing in small groups outside Burger King, waiting for someone to tell us what to do. Sometimes I didn't know what the plan was and no one was picking up their phones, so I'd wander over to Broadway by myself, walking back and forth every ten minutes or so, looking for someone I knew and trying to look like I was going somewhere else, like it was just an accident I'd happened by.

Eventually, as the sun set, dozens of kids would start streaming in, walking downtown from the crosstown M86 stop or uptown from the Tasti D-Lite, calling out to each other to see what the plan was—because in the time before cell phones you actually had to stop into places to find out what was going on—and then using the pay phone on the corner to page friends who hadn't shown up yet. There was a beeper code for "meet at Burger King," but I can't remember what it was.

When we'd gathered a big enough group, we'd wander through Central Park, head over to Andy's Deli to try to convince the homeless guy who hung out outside to buy us some St. Ides or over to the East Side to sit on someone's front stoop, and then usually end up sitting in the grass outside the Met after night fell, our backs against the slanting glass wall of the Egyptian exhibit, doing our best to get into trouble but mostly only playing game after game of "I Never."

That summer, a girl named Hannah seemed like the center of it all. She had long dark-brown bangs, wore glitter eye makeup and perfect bell-bottoms and her hair in two buns on top of her head, and was best friends with the boy I had decided that I was in love with for the moment. She seemed comfortable in a way that I wanted to be so badly; I never could figure out how to be at rest with myself with too many people around—especially people who I very much wanted to think I wasn't even thinking. About anything.

For a while, it felt like the answer to the way I felt might be something as small as the shade of my lipstick, or the shape of my jeans. If I could find a pair of bell-bottoms just like Hannah's, I thought, maybe I could trick them—and then trick myself—into thinking I wasn't just tolerated, but rather *necessary*. That they should call *me* from the pay phone to let me know that everyone was hanging out, we're all here, *you should come.*

I know: lots of teenagers do things like this. Drink things they shouldn't in places they shouldn't, date people they shouldn't. Push boundaries. "Act out." Except it wasn't enough for me. And later—much later—I realized that whatever I had been looking for in high school, I hadn't gotten yet.

The trend—or so I hear—is to get all your Wild out in college, and then to move on to a life of respectable adulthood complete with things like employment and responsibilities, but what I did instead was the reverse. I went to Harvard, and college was such a busy, full time for me that I spent my four years there being way less experimental than your average college student (or so I hear). I studied behavioral biology, went to sleep early for two nights before every exam, and enrolled in 8:30 a.m. classes because they were the best ones and were never full. And then I graduated, moved out to Hollywood to continue the acting career that I'd begun in high school, and went completely off the rails.

It was pretty much the kinds of things you might expect from a young actress who moves out to Los Angeles not really knowing anyone and gets an apartment right off of the Sunset Strip, within walking distance of the Viper Room and the Chateau Marmont and Miyagi's, a half sushi restaurant, half club with a confusingly cheap two-for-one drink special list. But going out way, way too much and way, way too late was only part of it. Mostly, it came down to this:

I always wanted to be the person who people called—who people didn't just tolerate, but *wanted there*. And for a while, in Los Angeles, it finally felt like I was, because I surrounded myself with people whose flawed priorities were perfectly aligned with my own. I was so unhappy during that time, so empty and confused and directionless, but that one thing that I'd always wanted—a phone that constantly rang with people wanting me to come out, come hang, *come be with us*—I had.

Except, more and more, I realized that the world that I had made myself so necessary to wasn't nearly as wonderful as I'd felt like it was. My "best friends" were barely even acquaintances; all I knew about them, really, was their drink order and whether they were good at darts; wherever we were was usually too loud to let me find out much else. It was a lonely place, and not somewhere I wanted to continue living.

One morning not long after I moved back to New York City, Kendrick and I met up with my parents for a Saturday morning canoe ride up the Delaware River. I was exhausted. We'd gone out late, way too late, the night before, and when my alarm went off only a couple of hours after I had fallen asleep I should probably have called my parents and made some excuse or another why I couldn't make it, but the idea of missing out on a day that I would have loved so much just a few years earlier suddenly made me desperately, hopelessly sad. And so I went, and I fell asleep in the canoe, and I slept through the entire ride down the river and the entire drive home and missed the day anyway. A whole day that would have made me so happy: gone, just like that.

I spent a lot of time in the months before my husband and I decided to have a baby worrying that once we found out we were expecting I'd have to change. "Grow up." I worried that the identity I had built for myself as the girl who was always game for staying out until the sun came up, for being wild and exciting and *fun* would collapse like a house of cards . . . because that part of me had become much more than just a "part"—in my mind it had become everything, almost. I remembered that my definition of fun had used to include a huge rainbow of things from canoe trips to cream sodas, but over the years that rainbow had whittled down to only those things that happened late, late at night—so late that thinking about my life and where it was headed (which felt like nowhere) was the very last thing on my mind, if it was there at all. I wanted to go back to being someone who enjoyed an early morning ride down the river, but I didn't know if I could remember how.

I didn't just "want" my life to be different than it was; I knew it *had* to. And so I started, if not settling down, exactly, settling *in*. Sifting through the piles of things I had thought I liked but had turned out to be not quite as wonderful as I'd imagined, in search of what actually might make me happy.

I worried about settling down because I worried that what it meant was letting go of the reckless joy that I thought was the point of it all, that I thought my husband and I needed to maintain to have a life worth living. And then, early one October morning, our son was born, and what he brought with him was reckless joy like we'd never known. More than that, he did the opposite of taking away those things about us that we had thought made us *us*; instead, he stripped away the picture we had made in our minds of who we had thought we wanted to be and told us the truth, uncovering parts of our hearts long paved over with expectations built out of sand.

I used to hate seeing the sunrise, because what it meant was that I'd stayed up too late, that another day was about to be wasted. But now I saw what early morning looked like again, and this time I saw it while sitting in a rocking chair, holding a person I loved in the silence and waiting for the sun.

"Sunlight, sunlight baby
  We just let go of the night now slowly
  We won't dance, we won't sing, we won't talk
  We just gonna watch how it bends."

—Harlem Shakes, "Sunlight"

"People will say all kinds of things
  But that don't mean a damn to me
  'Cause all I see is what's in front of me
  And that's you."

—Yeah Yeah Yeahs, "Poor Song"

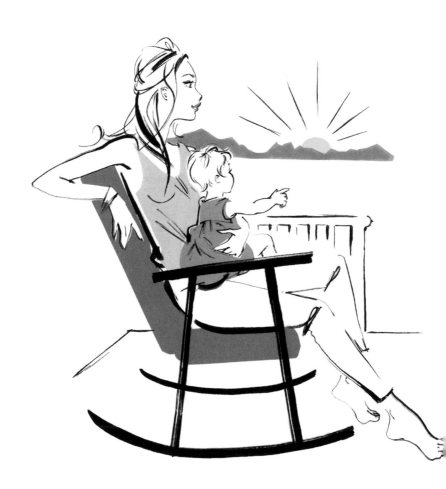

Come Away with Me?

ON THE DAY THAT I BROUGHT my son home from the hospital, I cried and cried. Partly because of the hormones and the postpartum depression, but mostly because it felt to me like we were children bringing a child home to a house that hadn't yet been built; a playground, not a refuge. The apartment building we lived in had hallways that still smelled of vomit from our neighbor's last party; there was a hole in the kitchen floor that our whiskey-swilling, William Blake–quoting superintendent "hadn't gotten around to" fixing for the past two years; the enormous heating pipe that clanged all night long ran straight through the part of the hallway that we'd designated as the nursery. When I put the baby down on the couch, I had to remember to put a pillow on his other side, because the whole place stood at a slight angle, and anything that you set down on a flat surface had a tendency to roll east.

I give a lot of lip service to the idea that you don't need to have a lot to have a baby; how preparation is important, but "having everything" isn't essential. How too much of a focus on "stuff" can actually get in the way, make it hard to see through all that stuff to what really matters.

I haven't always been able to follow my own advice.

Because having a baby—all the question marks and uncertainties and tectonic lifestyle shifts that come along with that kind of an undertaking—sends you to sea no matter what you've done to keep yourself on solid ground. And it can feel better, when you're out there on the waves, to know that you've built a good boat.

So when we found out we were expecting a second child, the thought that she'd have the things that our son hadn't had—a room of her own, a bedroom door, a station wagon with a pre-installed car seat—made me feel better. Safer. I painted her walls and folded her clothing and drove to Costco and stocked up on newborn-size diapers, planning out every detail of an arrival that I imagined would be the polar opposite of our son's: a calm homecoming of sleepy days and cozy nights and family movies under the covers of the king-size bed I'd bought so we'd have extra space in which to snuggle up with a baby, space we hadn't had the first time around. I pictured my daughter's first weeks of life spooling out in a slow, happy haze that I hoped would tell us that we'd done it: we had built a life for our children where they would be safe, where the steadiness of our days would let us see any dangers coming our way when they were still way out there on the horizon.

And then, two months before our daughter was set to arrive, when I was just starting to think about those last little details—packing up a hospital bag, hanging a mobile, which crib sheet to put on her mattress for her very first night sleeping in her very first bed—everything I had planned for changed. Just like that.

My husband was offered a three-month-long job across the country, a job too good to turn down, and so instead of spending the last weeks before our daughter's birth putting the finishing touches on her nursery and checking off those last few checkmarks left to be checked, we dropped off our dogs with a sitter and flew to California, our toddler holding a toy dinosaur in each hand, the flight attendant wedging a pillow under my lower back to "keep me comfortable" for the six-hour flight. We moved into a temporary housing complex with nothing more than whatever we could fit into three suitcases, planning to buy or borrow the rest. I worried about whether my son would be lonely without his friends, and whether I'd be able to find the small, sour mangos that were the only thing I wanted to eat at the end of my pregnancy at the local supermarket (which was where, exactly?). I wondered whether two car seats would fit into our tiny rental car once our daughter arrived, and stayed awake all night trying to think through everything that could possibly go wrong when we tried to fly back home at the end of the summer with a brand-new baby. I tried to see the dangers way out on the horizon, but the right-now was too choppy to see beyond tomorrow.

I didn't want to go. At eight months pregnant what I wanted was to rest, not to explore. I didn't want an adventure; I wanted to be in my own house, in my own bed, and to bring my baby home to her *home.*

And then I realized it; the thing that I think I knew already but needed to be reminded of: all the crib sheets and freezer-bagged meals and plans in the world don't mean a damn thing when what's really happening is the introduction of a brand-new life, with all the unplannable everythings that come along with a person who is not only part of you, but also a creation of his or her very own. Not a prize that you get as a reward for having "done a good job" these past nine months, but a launch pad for a story that has yet to be written.

You welcome a child into the journey that is your family's growing world, and there's something to be said for leaving some things open for discovery. For jumping in even when there might be a check mark or two left to be checked. For remembering that what this really is, is an *adventure*, and adventures can be imagined, but they cannot be contained.

A lot of what I write about is finding ways to keep doing the things you love when your family grows and your world shifts, about searching for what is exciting in what is scary. Because that exciting thing—that wonderful thing you never saw coming but that came anyway—is going to end up being what you remember most of all when it's over and in the past.

I write about these things, and our last-minute move was a reminder that I needed. A reminder to step away from the lists and the details and to stop pretending that I had control over the tide.

Most of all, though, our move reminded me of this: the adventures never have to stop. More than that: they can't. And you wouldn't want them to even if they could.

When I think about those first few weeks with our son, I don't remember the clanging pipe, the stained hallway, or the too-small bed. I don't remember the traffic or the four flights of stairs or the jackhammers that seemed to be running 24/7 right outside our bedroom window. I remember that my son's hair looked like baby duck fuzz, and that the skin on the soles of his feet matched the skin everywhere else on his body, because it had never been used. I remember sitting in my rocking chair with him, listening to classical music that I thought might calm him down but didn't and watching the first light of the sun come through our kitchen window. I remember that we began an adventure on the day that he was born, one that we only learned about as we lived it.

I'm scared of what lies ahead. Of course I am. But I'm also excited to tell my daughter, one day, that she was born in California, on a journey with her family that had only just begun.

. . .

*"You're always you, and that don't change,
and you're always changing, and there's nothing
you can do about it."*

—Neil Gaiman

Epilogue

· · · · · · · · · · ·

I'VE HEARD OF THOSE WOMEN who feel connected to the life growing inside them from the moment that life begins. Who lean back in their beds and talk to their unborn child, telling her all the things they can't wait to find out about her, all the things they hope she will see and do and learn and be. And when she is born, they recognize her instantly as a person they have always known.

While I waited for my daughter, I laid awake at night watching the skin of my stomach roll like the ocean, knowing that there was a person lying beneath but not "getting" it, not really. I tried to picture her tiny limbs pushing against my body, tried to imagine seeing her face, tried to imagine her growing into a person whom I could walk with in the woods by our house, but all I could see when I closed my eyes was the image from my latest what-size-is-your-baby-this-week e-mail newsletter, all umbilical cords and medical-textbook lines and bullet points telling me how big the fingers were or how quickly the neurons were developing.

And then my mind would turn to what to make for breakfast the next day, or when I'd be able to take in the car to get the windshield fixed, or whether my two-year-old son was happy, whether he was healthy, whether there were things that I could or should be doing for him that I wasn't. I worried about student loans yet to be paid, and whether my dog, who I could hear puttering around downstairs, was peeing on the corner of the couch again. I thought about the next day's deadlines, and the next time I'd be able to take a trip alone with my husband, how many years that trip was in the distance. I wondered whether strawberries were in season yet.

The baby wasn't real, and so what I thought about were the things that were; things right there next to me in the world, not tucked away in the dark in a place I couldn't even picture.

Yesterday, at just past eight o'clock in the morning, my daughter was born. I'm typing these words in a hospital bed with my sleeping baby next to me, my husband curled up on a couch with his head on a jacket, the beep-beep-beep of machines and my family's breaths the only sounds.

She's here with me, a person in the world. And I still don't know her—not really, not yet—but she is here, all butterfly-wing eyelids and dark swirls of hair and mystery. I don't know what she'll be like tomorrow, or the day after that, or five years from now, but what I know right now is that she is more real than I ever imagined during those long months of waiting, and that I can't wait to find out who she is, and the beauty she will bring.

In my twenties, I was so certain that the persona—the costume—that I had created for myself was made of cement and stone. I had a picture in my head of who I thought I was, and that picture seemed the realest thing of all, a thing that I should hold on to with an iron grip, lest something essential about me slip away. I was so scared that any changes that might happen in my life would change *me*.

I became a parent.

And I changed. Right back into the person I'd been all along.

And now I wouldn't change a thing.

Acknowledgments

. . . .

WRITING A BOOK while twenty million months pregnant and trekking back and forth across the country doesn't put one in the Zen-est of mindsets, so the first person I have to thank is my husband. Kendrick, thank you for being my biggest supporter, my partner in everything, and my best friend, for always ordering a meal that you think I'd like a bite of, and for teaching me how big of a difference a little listening can make.

Thank you to my management team at Digital Brand Architects—Karen Robinovitz, Kendra Bracken-Ferguson, Raina Penchansky, Maddy Gorin, and Ariana Pappas—and especially to Reesa Lake, who has been a cheerleader, a rock, an inspiration, and—most of all—a friend. Thank you also to my wonderful agent, Deborah Schneider at Gelfman Schneider.

To my editor and friend, Cindy De La Hoz, and the rest

of the publishing team at Running Press, especially Stacy Schuck, Chris Navratil, and Allison Devlin: having the opportunity to work with you twice in as many years has been such a pleasure. Thank you also to Sarah Pierson for bringing the pictures in my head to life with such thoughtfulness and skill, and to Jacqueline Bisset for the exceptionally beautiful artwork.

Making friends as a grown-up—forget about as a mother— is no easy feat, and I am so grateful for the women in my life. Francesca and Morgan, I am so fortunate that my children have you as examples of how remarkable women can be. Erin, thank you for always reminding me to be brave, in art and in life. Nadine, thank you for being right there with me (albeit virtually) the whole way through. Katie, Amy, Diana, Ella, Suzie, Penny, Tia—thank you for being the best, most supportive friends I could ever ask for, and for making our time on the East Coast so wonderful. I love you and will see you soon.

To my dear friend Daniel: I miss you and think of you and love you every day.

Huge thank-yous also go to the staff at the Lucille Packard Children's Hospital, who saw us through a tough transition and helped bring our beautiful daughter into the world, and to the Ramshackle Glam readers, who have always offered such an incredible support system. I am so thankful to you—all of you—for being a part of our life.

To River and Shea: There aren't words enough in a hundred books to tell you what you are to us, which is everything.

And finally, to Mom and Dad: I love you so much, and I get it now. Thanks for it all.